They
Don't Know
What's Wrong

Other titles by the same author

Complete Home Remedies
How to Live to 90

They Don't Know What's Wrong

DOES YOUR ILLNESS BAFFLE THE DOCTORS?

DR JAMES LE FANU

ROBINSON
London

Constable & Robinson Ltd
3 The Lanchesters
162 Fulham Palace Road
London W6 9ER
www.constablerobinson.com

First published in the UK by Robinson,
an imprint of Constable & Robinson Ltd 2001

A copy of the British Library Cataloguing in
Publication data is available from the British Library

ISBN 1-84119-305-4

Printed and bound in the EU

10 9 8 7 6 5 4 3 2

For the many readers of
The Daily Telegraph
without whom this book
could never have been written

Contents

Introduction

Modern medicine is a highly successful enterprise. Every day, each of Britain's 35,000 plus family doctors will see around 40 patients, adding up to nearly 9,000 consultations a year. They will issue more than 500 million prescriptions, or 10 per head of the population. Their hospital specialist colleagues will be equally busy, dealing with 10 million new patients a year and performing 5 million operations and procedures. The purpose of all this activity – obviously enough – is to cure or at least ameliorate one or other of the almost infinite number of ailments, both mental and physical, to which we are prone. It is also – initially at least – an exercise in problem solving. 'This person sitting before me in the consulting room tells me he has back ache (or chest pain, or diarrhoea),' a doctor says to himself. 'Now, which of the many possible explanations fits this case? And what test must I do in order to be sure of the diagnosis?'

This exercise in problem solving is not just a preliminary to treatment, but rather, as has been observed, 'an accurate diagnosis is 90 per cent of the cure,' for without first knowing what is wrong and making the correct diagnosis, it is unlikely that whatever treatment is proposed will put it right.

This diagnostic method has been compared to detective work where the sleuth piles up one vital clue after another in his relentless pursuit of 'Who dunnit?' For the most part, however, the diagnosis is staggeringly obvious. Indeed, it is not unusual nowadays for a patient to come to the surgery and tell the doctor what is wrong: 'My asthma is back again,' 'My ulcer is playing up,' 'I think I've got shingles.' And if the patient does not know, a few pertinent questions, a brief examination of the relevant part of the body, or a blood test or chest X-ray is all that is necessary to tell the difference between pleurisy and pneumonia, gallstones and gastritis.

So, the diagnosis is, for the most part, fairly straightforward. Indeed it could not be otherwise, for family doctors or hospital specialists would be simply overwhelmed by the vast tide of medical problems that sweep through the surgery door every day. And thanks to the wonder drugs discovered by the pharmaceutical companies and the skills of today's surgeons, there is usually something that can be done and the patient is hopefully grateful to have whatever is amiss resolved. This takes us back where we started – modern medicine is a highly successful enterprise.

This 'success' actually influences our expectations – we *expect* the doctor to know what is amiss (at times to the point of omniscience) and how to put it right, or at least how to direct us to someone who will know the answer. Doctors, too, expect there to be an answer and, when it is not obvious, become frustrated to the point of sometimes blaming the patient for their illness by suggesting their complaint is not real but imaginary – that it is 'all in the mind'.

It is against this background of the effectiveness of medicine which is so much greater than 50 years ago, and the expectation that it be so, that this book has been written. For, despite everything that has already been said, the unfortunate fact remains that doctors may *not* know what's wrong. There are, as might be expected, several possible reasons for this. They may not have listened closely enough to the patient's account of his symptoms, thus overlooking some important clue. Alternatively, they may have failed to do a vital test or misinterpreted its findings. They may have jumped to the wrong diagnosis and thus become frustrated because the appropriate treatment turns out to be ineffective. Then, medicine *can* be difficult, especially in the older age group who perhaps have two or three separate ailments where one set of symptoms muddy the waters, obscuring what would otherwise be a clear view of another set of symptoms. These reasons why they may 'not know what's wrong' will be elaborated further in the next chapter, but there is one further possible explanation that forms that core of this book and so will be considered here in some detail. 'They' may not know what's wrong because 'they' have never encountered the symptoms complained of, which indeed may be so bizarre and unusual that 'they' find it difficult to conceive what the explanation might be. By definition, these 'mystery syndromes' as I will call them are not common, but cumulatively the numbers of people experiencing one or other is likely to be quite considerable – as the thousands of letters I have received over the last two years amply confirm.

My interest in mystery syndromes started with a letter from a reader, Mr D.M. from Hythe in Kent, describing a set of symptoms which had apparently baffled no less than six different specialists. Almost every evening for a decade he had noticed 'an itchy tickling in the throat that induces an episode of convulsive coughing which ends in six huge sneezes'. This was accompanied by 'aching ears, a feeling in the nose and head as of a nasty cold, but no production of mucus'. Did I, he wondered, have any ideas as to what might be going on? I did not, but before I wrote back to tell him so, I mentioned his complaint in the weekly column I write for the *Daily Telegraph*. This, to my considerable surprise, elicited nearly 50 responses describing other instances of bizarre sneezing experiences and offering a fistful of possible explanations.

Two themes rapidly emerged from this correspondence. First, there is a lot more to sneezing than merely being an effective way of dislodging irritating particles from the nostrils. Sneezing might *seem* a simple and straightforward reflex – indeed most of the time it is – but there appear to be a variety of sneezing syndromes which never feature in the medical text books and about which most doctors are therefore unaware.

There would seem, for example, to be a form of inherited sneezing, as illustrated by the following account from Mr G.H. from the Wirral:

The sneezing fits happen more often than not in the early morning and are frequently a daily occurrence although I will sometimes go for a week without one. I sneeze violently between six and twelve times over a period of a couple of minutes. Interestingly my late father also suffered from sneezing fits – his were far more severe, often lasting for over ten minutes and leaving him like a wet rag. My brother has similar fits as do my two sons and also my two nephews.

Then there is a curious type of sneezing which appears to be triggered by an internal biological clock. Dr G.T. from Northamptonshire describes a 64-year-old accountant who otherwise enjoyed good health over the previous 30 years:

> These sneezing fits occur on average five times every week and can be quite alarming to those who do not know him. He usually sneezes nine times in rapid succession with no forewarning, no nasal irritation and little mucus; there is no eye watering or deafness. Even more curiously the attack almost invariably occurs within a few minutes of 9 p.m. and when he is abroad his nose sets itself to the new time zone within 24 hours!

The correspondence also revealed the remarkable range of often unlikely factors that can precipitate a bout of sneezing, including sudden changes of temperature ('if I get into the car which has been outside all night, in a few seconds I'll be off'); looking into bright lights or sunlight ('which can be hazardous on motorways'); sugar; white wine ('I have uncontrolled sneezing and runny nose within one to two hours or drinking half a bottle of cheap white wine. I might add I do not drink cheap white wine in my own house, but one cannot specify to one's friends what they should serve at dinner parties'); and newspaper print.

And what about the bouts of coughing and sneezing described by Mr D.M. from Hythe? Sir Donald Harrison, former president of the Royal Society of Medicine, wrote to say that his wife's sneezing had been found to be due to aspirin. Further enquiry revealed that Mr D.M. was taking a similar drug – ibuprofen – for control of his arthritis. Thus the mystery of Mr D.M.'s sneezing was solved, which was of course good news for him but also has much wider implications, because aspirin is now routinely prescribed to tens of thousands of people with circulatory problems such as angina or stroke. Hence the numbers whose 'mystery sneezing' might be due to aspirin is considerable.

I was intrigued by the variety and diversity of insights – most of which were completely new to me – generated by this one query. In retrospect, I now realise I had stumbled, quite by accident, on a novel – and very productive – method of coming up with answers for those whose doctors may 'not know what is wrong' – and for the following reasons.

The circulation of *The Daily Telegraph* is around 1.35 million, which gives it a readership in excess of 2 million, so if for the sake of argument, a quarter of those readers regularly peruse my column, that works out at a round figure of 500,000 in total. This contrasts with the mere 2,000 on the register of the average family doctor (of whom he will only ever see a quarter in any given year) or the around 1,500 new patients seen every year by the hospital specialists. Thus the range of medical symptoms and problems experienced by the readers of my *Daily Telegraph* column is greater by orders of magnitude than most doctors and specialists are likely to encounter in a lifetime. No matter how unusual or abstruse their medical problems, there will almost certainly be someone out there who has experienced something similar – or, even better, have an answer for it.

However, it took a letter from another reader before I fully realized how my column could act as a forum for ideas and suggestions about mystery syndromes. Mrs Hazel Pillatt from Milton Keynes wrote to say that while reading the Greek historian Herodotus, she had been struck by the parallel between the response to Mr D.M.'s sneezing enigma and Herodotus's description of the following Babylonian custom from the fifth century BC:

> They have no doctors, but bring their invalids out into the street, where anyone who comes along offers the sufferer advice on his complaint, either from personal experience or observation of a similar complaint in others. Anyone will stop by the sick man's side and suggest remedies which he has himself proved successful

in whatever the trouble may be, or which he has known to succeed with other people. Nobody is allowed to pass a sick person in silence; but everyone must ask him what is the matter ...

This Babylonian custom, she suggested, could readily be transferred into the twentieth century, by courtesy of my column. The following week, I cited Herodotus's quotation and suggested that those like Mr D.M., whose symptoms had baffled the specialists, should submit a brief description of their ailment which could then be published in the hope that others might be in a position 'to suggest remedies that had proved successful in whatever the trouble may be'.

Nothing could have prepared me for the scale and nature of the response. I think of myself as being a well-informed and knowledgeable family doctor, but the diversity of symptoms submitted was quite literally a revelation; not only were most completely new to me, it was difficult to conceive what their explanation might be. The verdict was inescapable – my medical knowledge was much less comprehensive than I realized, and so was that of my fellow doctors who, as the correspondence revealed, had been unable to come up with a satisfactory explanation for these mystery syndromes despite investigations too numerous to mention and consultations with many different specialists.

It might be thought that the failure to establish a diagnosis meant that frequently there was indeed nothing wrong, and that the readers afflicted by these mystery syndromes must be hypochondriacal or neurotic, expressing their mental unhappiness in a bizarre array of bodily symptoms. But this was definitely not the case. The symptoms recounted by readers were undoubtedly authentic, as was made clear not just by the manner in which they were recounted, but the way they were independently confirmed by others who had had similar experiences. Further, it soon emerged that the mystery syndromes were not quite as random and inexplicable as first appeared, rather they could be seen to fit into one of a variety of fairly well-defined categories. This will be discussed in more detail in the next chapter.

The correspondence revealed another important matter

which needs to be better appreciated. Those unfortunate enough to find that they are one of those whose doctors don't know what's wrong are caught in a most invidious situation. They obviously have to contend with the physical discomfort of their symptoms, for which, in the absence of an accurate diagnosis, no effective remedy is available. Further, the doctor's failure to find the cause of the complaint can also be psychologically very taxing. They have to live with the fear that whatever the explanation might turn out to be (and there is always the expectation that sooner or later someone will get to the bottom of it) will turn out to be quite serious. This is compounded by apprehension about what *might* happen in the future, as all those questions that patients might naturally wish to ask – How long will this last? When will I feel better? – will necessarily go unanswered. Then, as if this were not bad enough, they have to deal with the scepticism, or indifference, of doctors who are unable to put a label on their symptoms and who convey the impression – wittingly or not – that they are illusory. They get caught up in the wearisome rigmarole of modern medicine – yet more investigations, yet more referrals – and by the time they are seated in the consulting room of the umpteenth specialist, there is a strong sense of going through the motions when no one has any confidence that there might be a satisfactory outcome.

I sincerely hope that some at least of those who purchase this book will find an answer to their problem – and with it an end to such uncertainty. That said, I must conclude with a caveat, which I hope will be readily understood. The contents of this book are concerned not with what is known, but with what is unknown or poorly understood. It does not deal with a well-established body of knowledge, but rather with some observations, experiences, anecdotes and inferences. Its purpose, therefore, is less to 'provide answers', and more to act as a source of hints as to where to look further.

I scarcely need add that I would more than welcome any comments readers may have. Perhaps they recognize one or other of the mysteries in this book, or have some insights they would like to pass on. Or perhaps they have a mystery of their own that does not feature. Either way, please let me know.

1
'They Don't Know What's Wrong': An Overview

There is no nook or cranny of the body that cannot now be scrutinized. The shiny black endoscope transmits back to the viewer's eye the innermost recesses of the stomach and colon; the pulse sound waves of the ultrasound machine elicit echoes from deep within the pelvis; while CT and MRI scanners illuminate – with haunting clarity – the deepest structures of the brain enclosed within the skull. Modern techniques of chemical analysis achieve the same level of precision, capable of measuring every protein, enzyme or mineral in the bloodstream, in virtually infinitesimally low concentrations.

This diagnostic firepower is certainly impressive but the question posed by this book is why, nonetheless, may the doctor still 'not know what's wrong'? There would seem to be three main reasons. The first is human error – some important clue has been overlooked, or the wrong tests have been taken, or the right tests have been done but their results have been misinterpreted. Secondly, the cause of the medical problem may lie beyond the power of even the most sophisticated of diagnostic techniques to identify. The CT images of the brain can be almost supernaturally lucid, but they can still only identify defects that are visible to the human eye. If the source of the ailment lies at a more microscopic level in a single nerve or bundle of nerves, the scan will fail to detect it. And thirdly, the medical problem may be so novel or infrequent, or indeed so bizarre, as to fall outside the experience of most doctors and so they are unable to conceive what the explanation *might* be. Sophisticated tests notwithstanding, effective medical diagnosis is based, above all, on the recognition of *patterns* of symptoms which, when combined together, point to one illness rather than another.

It is simply not practicable to explore the full ramifications of these three reasons why doctors may not know what's wrong, but it is helpful briefly to outline the logical process by which both GPs and specialists do establish a diagnosis, the better to see the possible pitfalls. The family doctor's main priority is to pick out from the tide of problems that sweep through his surgery every day the serious ones, whose causes need to be clarified and which may need to be referred onward for a specialist opinion. The specialist's responsibility is to make a definitive diagnosis and define it accurately enough so that the best treatment can be decided on.

Both, however, rely on the three strands of the diagnostic process to elucidate what is going on: a history of the complaint, a physical examination and appropriate investigations.

I. THE HISTORY

The history is much the most important. The doctor, by asking *exactly* what is complained of, what brings it on and what relieves it, gets his patient to draw a picture of what is happening. With the help of years of experience, this allows him to recognize the characteristic pattern of symptoms of most illnesses that has already been alluded to.

There are, for example, dozens of different causes of headache and it would clearly be impossible to consider each possible explanation one by one. How does he, almost blithely, dismiss so many different possibilities and, hopefully, plump for the right explanation? Firstly, and obviously, headaches are a common feature of many illnesses – viral infections such as the flu, nervous disorders, blocked sinuses and so on. In each of these, however, there will always be further additional symptoms which focus the doctor's attention on which possibilities should be pursued. If there are none, this points to one or other of several types of primary headache – such as migraine, tension and cluster headaches. These can only be differentiated by fastidious attention to the details – which part of the head is involved, what is the nature of the pain, what brings it on, how long does it last, what relieves it? Some with a headache are not happy until they have had a brain scan to make sure they do not have a brain tumour. This is actually the last thing they need, as it will almost certainly distract attention from the much more important task of eliciting a comprehensive account of the complaint, which is required to make a correct diagnosis. The absolute importance of a proper history is well illustrated by the description from neurologist Dr Nick Fox of his dealings with a deaf mute woman whose almost continuous headaches of 40 years had been misattributed to 'migraine':

The situation was virtually impossible. Each question took several minutes to go through the interpreter, back and forth between husband and patient and then back to me. 'Her headache had been present for over 40 years, since the age of ten, was getting worse, was present all the time and the treatments do not work and no one listens or cares.' The gesticulating of hands around the head suggested 'pain all over'.

Only half listening I leafed through her voluminous hospital notes. She had been seen by several specialists and been investigated extensively. She had been tried on various treatments with little effect and had had side-effects with everything. I knew I had failed to understand her and her headache. She knew too. I increased the dose of her migraine treatment and weakly said these things took time and made her another appointment.

When I saw her again she was obviously no better. Her husband was sullen and glowering. She was tearful and handed me a note about how nothing had worked. It dawned on me I had not thought of conducting the interview with notes and diagrams. Slowly and laboriously she 'drew' her headache for me – it was continuous but fluctuated in severity. It was always left sided and never crossed the mid line. She had previously considered suicide because of the pain. None of the migraine treatments had helped. The history now sounded like *hemicrania continua* in which case the headache should respond to indomethacin. She agreed to try it.

Four weeks later she looked transformed. She handed me a note explaining her pain was better that it had been for 40 years. She had missed one dose of indomethacin and her pain had returned with a vengeance. A year on she remains nearly painfree.

It is scarcely necessary to labour the obvious point. It was only when Dr Fox overcame the communication difficulties and asked her to describe the precise characteristics of her headache that the diagnosis became clear and in doing so that it was of a type that uniquely and consistently responds to only one drug – indomethacin.

The moral is clear enough. As in life, so in medicine: the truth lies in the details – and the more detail the better. Every little particle of information counts, as is shown by another account of a 67-year-old man who sought medical attention for earache.

For several years a 67-year-old man had complained of intermittent pain in the left ear initially described as a feeling of pressure. Ear and nose examination was normal. Subsequently the ear pain became incapacitating. It was provoked by cold weather, physical exertion and emotion and was relieved after a brief rest. Since these provocative factors were similar to those frequently encountered in angina, he was referred for an exercise test which indicated reduced working capacity due to recurrence of the severe ear pain. He was considered for coronary bypass and coronary angiography revealed narrowing of the main coronary artery. Three weeks later while waiting for his operation he died suddenly from a heart attack.

The crucial detail here, of course, is that the earache was closely related to exertion and though of course the familiar recognizable pattern of chest pain on exertion is readily diagnosed as angina, the same diagnosis almost always applies to any symptoms associated with exertion. If the many doctors he had consulted over several years had appreciated this a bit earlier and instigated the appropriate investigations leading to a bypass operation, his life would almost certainly have been saved.

2. THE PHYSICAL EXAMINATION

Physical examination has in recent years largely been displaced by modern diagnostic techniques which are both more definitive and accurate. When it comes to knowing what is going on in the lungs, the stethoscope cannot compete with the chest X-ray.

There are times, of course, when the physical examination is invaluable, as in someone complaining of deafness. Here a quick glance down the eardrum will readily distinguish between the three main causes – wax, glue in the middle ear (as shown by bulging of the eardrum) and, if neither of these signs are present, the culprit is almost certainly age-related hearing loss, or presbyacusis. The decline in the significance of physical examination in making a diagnosis means it is unlikely to be, by itself, the explanation for why 'they don't know what's wrong' – with the following exception. Physical examination is almost invariably focused on the part of the body from which the symptoms apparently originate, which can mean that some important sign elsewhere in the body is overlooked.

This is illustrated by the account of a 34-year-old man, the cause of whose cough – which he had had for 15 years – only emerged when it was noted to synchronize with an irregularity of the heartbeat.

> He was disturbed and despairing because despite extensive investigation no cause had been found. The previous year the episodes had become much more frequent, lasted longer and occurring almost every day and at night. Physical examination was normal except for frequent dry coughs and an irregular pulse. While we were feeling the patient's pulse we noticed his cough always occurred when his pulse missed a beat which an ECG showed was due to premature contraction of the atrium of the heart. This was treated with beta blockers, the heart rate returned to normal and the attacks of coughing decreased from many times daily to no more than a couple of episodes a week lasting only a few seconds.

Again the point hardly needs emphasizing. For 15 years, his doctors had focused their attention on his lungs which was the natural place to look for the source of his cough. The association of that cough with his irregular heartbeat (both presumably mediated by irritation of the same nerve) may be unusual, but could only have been detected by the doctor observing the pattern of his coughing while feeling his pulse.

3. INVESTIGATIONS

Modern medicine has come to rely on sophisticated diagnostic investigations to find out what is wrong for the very good reason that they can illuminate in extraordinary detail the innermost parts of the body that previously could only be felt, palpated, or listened to from the outside. The trouble is that these tests can be almost too easy to do, so 'I think we should do a few more tests' can easily become a substitute for thinking. Nor, of course, are they infallible. They can reveal abnormalities that subsequently turn out to be irrelevant, or, as already observed, they can be normal despite the presence of disease. These are known as 'false positive' and 'false negative' tests respectively.

We start with the false negative as illustrated by a man in his mid-70s whose complaints of loss of weight and nocturnal back pain are strongly suggestive of a tumour of the pancreas. The appropriate investigation – a CT scan of the abdomen – is however reported as normal. The most obvious diagnosis having been considered and excluded, the doctors' attention then turns to other possibilities, which not surprisingly fail to clarify what is going on. Months elapse before the patient seeks a second opinion and the specialist, noting the persistence of the original symptoms, suggests the scan be repeated. By now, however, the tumour is only too obvious but regrettably has spread so far in the intervening months that surgical operation is no longer possible.

The reverse situation arises with the false positive tests. Here, for instance, a woman in her mid-50s with low back pain consults an orthopaedic surgeon, who advises that the best way of sorting out what is going on is to have an MRI scan. This is duly performed and reveals a protruded disc pressing on a nerve which is removed at operation. The woman's back pain persists as before, for which the only possible reason must be that the protruding disc was not the source of her original symptoms. This unfortunate situation is not unusual. Indeed, when a Californian radiologist had the subversive idea of doing MRI scans of the lower spine on 100 people with no symptoms of back pain, she found 66 separate abnormalities – protruded discs, arthritis of the joints – which, had they occurred in somebody with symptoms, would almost certainly have resulted in an operation.

This schematic outline of the diagnostic process highlights two of the explanations for why they may not know what's wrong. There is the sin of *omission*, the failure to ask the right questions, examine the right part of the body or do the right test. Consequently, a vital clue is lost and that which should have been made clear remains clouded in obscurity. And then there is the sin of *commission*, where an erroneous diagnosis is made on the basis of a less than thorough history or an over-interpreted abnormal investigation. The truth is then overlooked, as the doctor gets sidetracked by the red herring of a misleading diagnosis and long periods can elapse before someone says, 'Hang on a minute, let's go back to the beginning and see what's really going on here.' There is no easy way of knowing whether one or other of these reasons accounts for the fact that 'they don't know what's wrong' – but the following observations are relevant.

Firstly, modern diagnostic techniques *are* very good – that is, one should expect them to be able to identify the cause of symptoms and if they are unable to do so, it is fair to assume – at least initially – that one or other of these sins of omission or commission are responsible. The solution here is to seek a second opinion, as a fresh look at an old problem frequently works wonders.

Secondly, modern methods of treatment are also highly effective and so one should expect that whatever treatment is recommended should at least ameliorate the symptoms. If it fails to do so, again, the possibility must be considered that the doctor is barking up the wrong tree, pursuing a red herring, or whatever other metaphor is preferred. By definition, the 'right' treatment will not work for the 'wrong' diagnosis, and in this situation a reevaluation of the problem is called for.

The time has now come to turn attention in rather more detail to the third of our possible explanations for why 'they don't know what's wrong', where the symptom complained of is so unusual or falls so far outside the doctor's experience that he has difficulty in envisaging what the problem might be. The description of these 'mystery syndromes' is the main concern of this book, and the invaluable contribution of the readers of the *Daily Telegraph* in clarifying them has been discussed in the Introduction. They are so numerous and diverse as to suggest there must be a lot of people out there unaware there may indeed be an explanation for their unusual symptoms.

These syndromes can be so unusual or bizarre as not to conform to any recognizable pattern of illness and consequently they defy the attempts of numerous specialists and batteries of investigations to determine their cause. The doctors are mystified and not infrequently give the impression that the symptoms cannot therefore be 'real', but must be all in the mind – the physical expression of an over-active imagination. Their reality, however, cannot be in doubt. Not only are they frequently independently confirmed by others, but their specificity and particularity – and the discomfort and suffering they cause – are unquestionably authentic.

Their diversity notwithstanding, it is possible to identify a pattern to these mystery syndromes' where for the most part they can be seen to fit into one or other of the following categories.

The Rare But Recognized

The pattern of symptoms in this common source of mystery syndromes has indeed been described at some time in the past but is so unusual that most doctors will have never encountered it.

(i) *Taste-induced (gustatory) sweating* 'My main trouble is that over the last few months whenever I come into contact with an atmosphere where food is being fried I immediately start to sweat profusely, but only on the face and scalp.'

This phenomenon of taste (or smell) induced sweating was first described in 1923 by neurologist Lucie Frey, and indeed it is sometimes known as Frey's syndrome. It is presumed to be due to 'inappropriate' connections between the olfactory (smelling) nerve and the sweat glands.

(ii) *Migrating skin sensitivity* 'It all started with flu-like symptoms and then progressed to sensitivity of the skin on different parts of the body – thighs, armpits, upper arms, shoulders and midriff. The sensitivity remained in one area for a few weeks before moving on to another area. The sensitivity is to light touch only. Heavy pressure has no effect, in fact gives relief.'

The migrating nature of this skin sensitivity is strongly suggestive of the condition known as Wartenberg's neuritis, where 'stretching' the sensory nerves under the skin causing pain and numbness.

(iii) *Mouth blisters* 'I suffer from massive blood blisters on my tongue caused by simple things such as a rough edge on an apple, biscuits, toast, etc.'

This is a rare chronic blistering disease known as benign mucosal pemphigoid which effects the mucous membranes of the mouth and genital tract. Further well-recognized precipitants include hot drinks and ginger biscuits.

The Functional

The problem here is some abnormality of the functioning of an organ – the classic example being irritable bowel syndrome, where the symptoms of colicky pain and constipation or diarrhoea stem from the incoordination of the function of the muscles in the wall of the bowel. Thus though the symptoms are real enough, there is nothing 'to see' when the relevant part is examined or investigated.

The same principle applies to the intermittent episodes of pain and difficulty in swallowing due to spasm of the muscles around the oesophagus:

My problem has happened about half a dozen times – always when I have been dining in a restaurant. When the meal is placed in front of me I eat the first two or three mouthfuls but then my digestive system seizes up and I suddenly find I cannot eat or drink and my mouth fills with saliva. I then have to retire to the loo. The only solution seems to make myself vomit and then to try to get rid of the pockets of air which seem to be trapped under the food.

Ageing

The body is so wondrous in the infinite complexity of its working parts that, regrettably, there are virtually an infinite variety of ways for them to go wrong with the passage of years. The common age-related medical problems such as arthritis, cataracts and furred-up arteries are readily recognizable, but many others are less so. They not infrequently mimic other conditions and, as with the functional disorders mentioned above, investigation fails to reveal an underlying cause, leaving ageing as the only possible explanation.

(i) *Watery eye* 'When the weather is cold and/or windy my eyes water very badly. I am 77 years old and still enjoy playing golf two or three times a week but the pleasure can sometimes be spoilt by my inability to see the ball clearly enough. Neither my doctor nor optician have offered any suggestions.'

There are two well-recognized causes of watering eye – weakness of the muscles of the eyelid, or blockage of the duct through which the tears drain away. When, however, the eyelids are fine and the duct is not blocked, then watery eye is likely to be due to an age-related defect of the tear film.

(ii) *Drooling* 'There is a constant trickle of saliva from the right-hand side of my mouth and I can feel drops forming on my chin. Mopping this up constantly is beginning to mark my skin which is becoming red and scaly.'

Drooling is a symptom of Parkinson's disease where there is a reduced ability to swallow saliva, and may occur in neurological disorders such as cerebral palsy. When, however, it is – as here – a solitary symptom, ageing is the likely cause.

The Sensory Nerves

Bizarre sensory symptoms are a recurring source of mystery syndromes which are presumably due to a malfunctioning of the sensory nerves, which can be responsible for a wide variety of unpleasant sensations.

(i) *Sweet/salty taste* 'I have a horrid salty taste in my mouth about which I have consulted my family doctor three or four times to no avail. It seems to get worse at different times of the month and the edges of my tongue can feel quite sore although there is nothing to see. It is most unpleasant.'

(ii) *Burning feet* 'I have a mixture of pain and burning sensation on the soles of both feet. I get good relief when standing and therefore putting the weight of my body on the feet so there is not much of a problem during the day. The main trouble is at night where the pain either stops me from going to sleep properly or wakes me up every couple of hours. So now I have insomnia, or at any rate difficulty in sleeping. It has become most troublesome.'

These abnormalities of sensation have been compared to the 'phantom pains' following leg amputation where the sensory nerves generate garbled or distorted messages. They can be very difficult to treat.

Migraine

Migraine – without a headache – is responsible for several mystery syndromes. The classic migraine headache is due to spasm of the blood vessels within the skull – first constriction, followed by dilation. When this same migrainous phenomenon affects other blood vessels in the abdomen or the balance mechanism in the middle ear, it will predictably enough result in a different set of symptoms.

(i) *Abdominal migraine* 'Initially my husband is irritable and hungry. He begins to sniffle as though he has a cold and feels very tired. By the next day he is queasy, quite often with a temperature and for several hours vomits a great deal of bile. He is really poorly but never experiences any pain. These attacks last for up to 30 hours and after a day to restore his strength, he is fit and well again. We have lost count of the number of fruitless visits to specialists.'

(ii) *Migrainous vertigo* 'A 71-year-old woman reported recurrent dizziness over the past 50 years. Her episodes were characterized by a 'swimming sensation' in her head along with nausea and vomiting, difficulty with concentration and a feeling of unsteadiness when attempting to walk. During an attack she experienced a marked sensitivity to movement and preferred to lie completely still. Her dizzy spells typically lasted from 12 to 15 hours. The frequency was about once every three weeks. She also reported severe headaches every one or two years since her late 20s. Her maternal aunt had similar occurrences of dizziness and her son had migraine.'

'Alternative' Medicine

One of the recurring themes described by those afflicted by mystery syndromes is how, following numerous unhelpful specialist opinions and umpteen investigations, they seek help from an 'alternative' practitioner – who immediately knows what's wrong. The reason for this curious state of affairs is that mainstream medicine refuses to recognize certain types of 'alternative' explanations for illness, and wrongly dismisses them as quackery. Thus those consulting a gut specialist will have numerous investigations to visualize the internal lining of the gut, but the possibility that food sensitivity or allergy might be responsible for their symptoms is simply ignored. Similarly, most doctors know little or nothing about those conditions for which osteopaths or chiropractors, with their skilled manipulative techniques, can diagnose promptly and treat efficiently.

(i) *Interstitial cystitis and food sensitivity* Interstitial cystitis is one of several ailments that closely mimic some other straightforward medical condition – in this case the bladder infection cystitis. The symptoms of pain on urination and increased frequency are the same, but there is no evidence of an infection.

The cause is unknown, but there is no doubt that food sensitivity can be responsible, as the following account reveals:

> It took me three years to find out the problem was acid of any kind: citrus juice, wine, brandy, sherry and gin and tonic, vinegar, most fruits and even marmalade. The reason it took me so long was that the various items took different times to affect the bladder, for instance it was 36 hours after drinking wine before it affected me and it took three days to clear through; orange juice reacted almost immediately but the effect was over within hours. I took my story to my current doctor but it was obvious he didn't believe me and it was a great relief to find another sufferer – believe it or not – at a cocktail party. I was able to believe I wasn't imagining 15 years of misery (walking downstairs was uncomfortable, a car ride was awful and sex was hell!).

(ii) *Sore tongue and food allergy* A persistently sore tongue, often with a 'scalded' feeling, can understandably be very distressing. The cause is generally deemed to be unknown but, as the following account reveals, the culprit can be allergy to food preservatives:

> For several years I suffered intermittently from a tongue which was either sore at the tip and edges or felt 'scalded'. Eventually I discovered I was allergic, among other things, to a group of chemicals (benzoates) which are widely used as food preservatives. 'Sore tongue' sufferers can start to help themselves by avoiding processed foods and drink as much as possible – particularly those items which are kept after opening for any length of time. My tongue is now comfortable most of the time, but occasionally the problem recurs if I have made an unwise choice when eating out.

The Uncommon Cause of a Common Condition

The family doctor would never be able to deal with his, on average, 40 patients a day were it not that luckily most medicine is fairly straightforward and the cause of the majority of complaints readily elicited. This expectation of an obvious explanation is so strong that, when it is not fulfilled, the possibility that the cause may be some other more unusual problem may not be considered and so the patient's symptoms will go undiagnosed.

(i) *Ear pain and acid reflux* Acid reflux is, to put it mildly, a most unlikely cause of pain in the ear – but it can happen, though as in this account, it took four years before the correct diagnosis was made.

> An 82-year-old proprietor of an old people's home complained of recurrent painful episodes in the right ear for the previous four years. It initially occurred at regular intervals but had become more frequent during the previous six months, occurring every morning and recurring variably late in the day. The pain was described as a severe deep-seated ache. He tried various analgesics, deriving some benefit, but had gained complete relief about 30 minutes after taking antacids. His wife, who accompanied him, reported that two doctors curtly dismissed the idea that antacids could relieve his earache. At times he regurgitated a bitter tasting fluid into his mouth and a barium meal examination identified a hiatus hernia. I explained the pain probably arose from stimulation of the vagus nerve and medication with an acid suppressant at night resulted in no further pain in the ear.

(ii) *Sciatica and an aberrant artery* There are few more clear-cut and dramatic symptoms than the powerful shooting pain down the leg caused by pressure on the sciatic nerve as it emerges from the lower back – commonly referred to as sciatica. The following case explains how the failure to respond to standard treatment indicates the possibility of an uncommon cause of a common condition.

> A 33-year-old man was referred to hospital with an eight-year history of right sciatic pain exacerbated by physical activity. He was an enthusiastic skier, trekker and soccer player and his sciatica caused him severe physical and psychological distress. He sought several opinions and had undergone numerous investigations – none of which had shown any abnormality. Neither physiotherapy nor anti-inflammatory and muscle-relaxant drugs provided any relief. A neurosurgeon was asked to explore the sciatic nerve and at operation there was a loop of the inferior gluteal artery compressing the sciatic nerve. The artery and nerve were carefully

separated and a patch was interposed between. Following surgery the patient's pain cleared completely. When seen a year later he had had no recurrence.

The Scientifically Inexplicable – The Kundalini Serpent

The success of Western medicine is grounded in the basic sciences of anatomy, physiology and biochemistry. But what if there were, in addition, 'hidden' forces or channels – like those through which acupuncture is claimed to work? Might they account for some mystery syndromes?

> For the last ten years I have had the following symptoms which always happen in bed. They start as a tingling beginning in my feet, slowly intensifying, it works its way up to my head where it 'blasts off' with a whirling dizziness. It is something like an orgasm but considerably more violent. I am then perfectly normal again. Occasionally I have had the whole episode for a second time but that is very rare.

A reader comments:

> This sensation is one which many would envy. It is a rising energy up the spine of the Kundalini serpent, a practice long known and understood from ancient times in India. Many mystics go into deep meditation to encourage this experience. I experienced a 'triple rising' some years ago without knowing what it was. I am not a New Age nut but a 70-year-old grandmother of the old school.

'True' Mysteries

There remain a considerable number of 'mystery syndromes' for which a satisfactory explanation was not forthcoming, which may well be being described for the first time.

(i) *Flat beer syndrome* 'When I drink a pint of beer it goes flat in the glass immediately. When the glass is refilled it immediately loses its head – even before I have touched it. My urine is frequently oily. I also note that if I drink red wine an oily film forms on the top.

(ii) *Chinese burn* 'I am a 56-year-old woman who for the last four years has had pins and needles and sharp stabbing pains in my hands and feet. Over the years these have progressed to include my face and scalp. The sensation is not particularly a numbness, more a Chinese burn.'

In summary, this book I hope will prove useful for many of those whose doctors 'don't know what's wrong'. The answer may well lie within its pages – or if not, readers should get some sense of which of the various categories their mystery syndrome may belong to. There will, at the least, be some reassurance in knowing that they are, after all, not alone.

2

The Sense Organs: Eyes, Ears, Nose and Mouth

The Eyes

The eye is very similar to a camera – with two further and distinct advantages. Firstly, the tears – together with the blinking of the eyelids – protect the cornea and keep it moist. Secondly, the movement of the muscles at the back of the eye can track a moving image as it passes across the field of vision. There are, inevitably with so beautiful and complex a structure, many things that can go wrong to cause pain or loss of vision and the optician or eye specialist usually has little difficulty in establishing the diagnosis.

This section is concerned with a handful of conditions for which there may not necessarily be a satisfactory explanation.

WATERY EYES

There are two reasons for watery eyes – either the blinking muscles of the eyelid which act as a pumping mechanism moving the tear film across the eyeball may be defective, or the duct through which the tears drain away may become blocked due to an infection or a small stone. Here the treatment involves putting right whatever is amiss, so if the eyelid muscle 'pump' is faulty, this can be repaired by tightening up the weaker muscles, while an obstruction by the tear duct can be relieved by a small operation. When, however, the eyelids are fine and the duct is not blocked, other possibilities must be considered.

Query 1 Mr I.L., a 77-year-old quantity surveyor from Esher, writes:
'*When the weather is cold and/or windy my eyes water very badly.* I am 77 years old and still enjoy playing golf two or three times a week, but the pleasure can sometimes be spoilt by my inability to see the ball clearly enough. Neither my doctor nor optician have offered any suggestions.'

Query 2 Mrs S.G. from Argyll writes:
'*I am blinded by tears the moment I open the front, or back, door in the morning.* Some days are worse than others. Tears fall as I bend to work in the garden and for a little while after I have come indoors. Visits to shops have a similar effect. I often have to assure people I am not crying as I fish in pockets for tissues to mop my eyes and nose.'

Comment There were two very useful suggestions:

Wrap-around Glasses

The excess tears may be an over-reaction to exposure to cold or wind.

♦ 'I am a golfer and my solution is to wear clear wrap-around cycling glasses. Though not completely wind-proof I am now able to walk directly into strong cold winds without the watery discomfort I had previously.'

♦ 'I suspect the cause may be cold wind getting 'trapped' between my spectacles and my eye. This must be a common problem for golfers as I read in a golf magazine that a side shield on the side of glasses protects golfers from excess lacrimation in wind and rain.'

Artificial Tears

It is possible, if certainly paradoxical, that watery eyes may be due to 'dry eyes'. This requires some understanding of the nature of the tear film itself, which consists of three layers: an outer fatty layer which is secreted by glands near the eyelashes; a middle aqueous layer that comes from the lacrimal gland and an inner mucus layer secreted by glands on the inner aspect of the eyelid. If, for some reason, the glands secreting the outer or inner layer of the tear film are defective, the tears will dry out and in response the lacrimal glands will over-compensate, producing an excess of tears.

♦ 'I was told by an ophthalmic consultant my watering eyes were due to dry eye(!!) He told me that the tear glands over-react to cure the problem and so produce watery eyes. I was prescribed artificial tears which did the trick.'

♦ 'I tried various eye drops to lubricate the eye without success, but as my optician told me a study was in progress using a high dose of cod liver oil, I thought I should try it. I limited my intake to the recommended daily dose and am pleased to report my eyes are much more comfortable.'

DRY/GRITTY EYES

The sensation of dry or gritty eyes can be induced by problems with any of the three layers of the tear film already described. Thus the outer fatty or liquid layer may be deficient due to disorders of the eyelid as can occur with skin conditions such as rosacea or blepharitis. The inner (mucus) layer may be deficient due to problems with the inner surface of the eyelid caused by certain skin conditions and vitamin A deficiency, resulting in drying up of the cornea. Much the most important cause of dry eye, however, is a defect in the production of the middle aqueous layer by the lacrimal glands. This is almost invariably associated with the condition known as Sjogren's syndrome (named after the Swedish ophthalmologist who first described it), where not only the eyes but also the nose and mouth can be affected.

Comment The obvious treatment is artificial tears to compensate for the defective functioning of the lacrimal glands.

- ♦ 'I use Hypromellose eyedrops during the day and sweet almond oil helps me through the night. Newer lubricants such as Visco tears and Gel tears have a longer duration of action and are equally effective.'
- ♦ An alternative approach is to prevent the tears that are produced from draining away through the tear duct as Dr Mark Wright describes: 'The outflow can be reduced temporarily by implanting gelatine rods or by cauterizing the tear duct. As 75 per cent of the tears drain through these ducts, the symptoms associated with moderately severe dry eyes may therefore be ameliorated.'

EYE PAIN

Virtually all pains in the eye are due to some problem in the eye itself, whose cause can usually readily be ascertained by an ophthalmologist. Where the cause is not apparent, then it is probable that the pain is coming from one or other of the several sensory nerves which supply the eye and surrounding structures.

The Needle in the Eye Syndrome

Neurologist Dr John Pearce from Hull points out that this rarely described 'pain with no name' is actually quite common but of unknown cause and difficult to treat:

This is *a vicious sudden stab of pain* experienced in one eye which lingers for a few seconds. It feels like a needle, knife or nail being driven deep into the eyeball. 'It is so severe if it didn't go so quickly I would scream,' one patient commented. For up to five minutes after there is a dull localized ache in the eye. It recurs several time during one day and may return irregularly for a few days before disappearing for weeks or months. There is no associated disturbance of vision or any other symptoms suggestive of migraine. The pain is far too brief to be considered a variant or cluster headache or trigeminal neuralgia. The nature of the pain itself precludes any sort of therapy as no tablet, inhalation or suppository could reach its target before the symptoms have spontaneously settled. Supportive therapy, now a much neglected art, is important; we doctors should show that we recognise the complaint and, not content just to *offer* reassurance, we should make sure we have secured it.

Cramp-like Pain at Night

Query Miss K.L. from Kent writes:

For over 30 years *I have had acute pain in my right eye which comes on only while I am asleep.* It is sharp and cramp-like which wakes me up and will not allow me to stay in bed. It has worsened throughout the years. At first it happened relatively frequently but now it wakes me every night. I have attended many hospitals, doctors and alternative therapists and tried many drugs, none of which have succeeded in any way at all.

Comment There was a single suggestion as to the possible cause of this distressing symptom.

Some 13 or 14 years ago I experienced identical symptoms – the pain in the eye was intense just as though someone had stabbed me. This happened several times over a year or two – enquiries of friends could not help. A visit to the optician could not give me an answer. Eventually I was referred to a specialist who came up with the answer which was Reis Buckler dystrophy which was caused by recurrent erosions of the cornea.

Tic Doloureux or Trigeminal Neuralgia

Query Retired nurse Mrs C.S. from West Sussex writes:

For quite a number of years I have had the following intermittent symptoms which occur possibly when I am overtired. They start with a *'tender' sensation to the lightest touch of my left eyelid and a 'sore' feeling on turning the eye.* This 'tenderness' progresses to the left side of the face, the gums, and the upper molars also feel tender. The symptoms disappear after about three days.

Comment This is a variation of the pain of trigeminal neuralgia, or tic doloureux arising from the facial nerve (see Facial Pain).

Four More Possible Causes of Eye Pain

♦ Pressure on the back of the head can produce a tender sensation which in turn reproduces or aggravates pain in the eye. Injection of the relevant nerves with a steroid and local anaesthetic brings substantial relief.
♦ The drug nifedipine, used for the treatment of raised blood pressure and angina, has been reported to be associated with eye pain.
♦ Visual display units may be associated with eye strain, but the evidence is disputed.
♦ Faulty movement of the jaw (the tempromandibular joint) has also been associated with eye pain (see Facial Pain).

Finally, an unsolved mystery: Mrs D.L. from West Sussex writes: 'For nearly 18 months now I have woken to find that *the corners of my eye (either side of the nose bridge) are smudged black as if they have been bruised.*'

The Ears

Our ears are the shape they are so they can channel sounds down the canal to the eardrum and, the better to do this, they grow in size over decades. This compensates for the gradual age-related decline in hearing – which is why those in their 70s and 80s have disproportionately large ears. Dr James Heathcote from Bromley measured the length of the external ear in 200 people between the ages of 30 and 93 and found a very clear gradient in size between the youngest and the oldest, from which he calculated that on average our ears grow at a rate of 0.22mm a year.

There are several mystery ear syndromes, most of which are related to the several different nerves that supply the outer and inner ear. They include nerves from the back of the neck (the cervical vertebrae), the facial nerve which conveys sensation from the face to the brain, the mandibular nerve which does the same for the jaw, and a branch of the vagus nerve that runs all the way down to the diaphragm.

PAINFUL EARS

Most cases of ear pain are due to infection or increased pressure behind the ear drum, both of which are easy to diagnose. But when the ear appears normal, several possibilities must be considered.

Arthritis of the Spine

Dr Tim Lamer from the Mayo Clinic in Rochester reports the case of a 51-year-old truck driver who presented with a five-week history of *pain in the ear lobe whenever he turned his head towards the right.*

> The pain was associated with intermittent numbness in the area behind the ear extending to the angle of the jaw reproduced by turning his head to the right and holding the position for several seconds. Cervical spine X-rays revealed extensive degeneration of the cervical spine and an injection with anaesthetic and steroid resulted in complete and sustained relief of his symptoms.

Malocclusion of the Jaw

The jaw joint, or tempromandibular joint – the smallest in the body – is believed by some doctors to be responsible for a variety of symptoms including impaired hearing, stuffy sensation in the ears, ear pain and tinnitus. The solution is a specially designed dental appliance, as described by Dr Elliot Alphers from Washington in a 62-year-old woman who had a 33-year history of *recurring episodes of sharp pain originating in front of her left ear and radiating down the left side of her neck.*

> Repeated dental, ENT and neurological examinations over the

years have been reported negative. She was found on examination to have crepitation of both tempromandibular joints. Mounted casts of the patient's dentition were then analysed and dental appliances fabricated. All symptoms disappeared within two weeks of the start of treatment. Jaw movements expanded to normal limits and all analgesics were discontinued.

Another reader comments:

I had ear pain for many years and went back and forth to my GP trying various options (including inhalers for my sinuses!). Eventually I was referred to an ENT specialist at London's St Barts Hospital who put his finger in my ear and asked me to bite. Immediately he recognized the problem and referred me to the dental department for a 'bite guard'. This is a soft plastic guard which fits over my lower teeth and very slightly relieves my 'bite' when I am asleep. After nine years of going to my doctor, the relief was tremendous with the right treatment!

Acid Reflux

The vagus nerve is the longest in the body, running all the way from the back of the brain down through the ear into the chest before terminating in the diaphragm. It is implicated – as described in Chest Syndromes – as a cause of a persistent cough and here Dr J.N. Blau of the National Hospital for Nervous Diseases describes its role in ear pain:

An 82-year-old proprietor of an old people's home complained of *recurrent painful episodes in the right ear* for the previous four years. Initially it occurred at irregular intervals but had become more frequent during the previous six months, occurring each morning and recurring variably late in the day and more so during the evening. The pain, described as a *severe deep-seated ache* was felt inside his right ear *radiating upwards and forwards towards the right temple*. He had tried various analgesics, deriving some benefit, but had gained complete relief about 30 minutes after taking antacids. His wife, who accompanied him, reported that two doctors had curtly dismissed the idea that antacids could relieve his ear ache.

At times he regurgitated a bitter tasting fluid into his mouth and a barium meal examination had identified a hiatus hernia. I explained the pain probably arose from stimulation of the vagus nerve and medication with the acid suppressant ranitidine 300mg at night resulted in no further pain in the ear or head.

ITCHY/BURNING EARS

Query 1 Mrs W.L., a retired civil servant from Bolton, writes:

> About two years ago I became aware of an *almost unnoticeable itch on the external part of my right ear as though a tiny mite was running about under the surface of the skin*. Over the months it has gradually got worse until it is now a deep-seated burning itch right down inside both my ears. Fortunately it is intermittent, otherwise it would have driven me mad, but never a day goes by without one or more bouts and sometimes it wakens me in the night. It leaves my ears and the side of my face down to the jawline feeling quite tender, with occasional prickling darts of pain.

Query 2 Mrs M.W. from Wigan reports: 'I have a *fiery burning sensation in and around my left ear*. Sometimes it is inside the ear, sometimes the part of the face just around the ear. My skin and ear do not feel warm and are not pink or red yet they burn fiercely.'

Comment Much the commonest cause of an itchy ear is an infection of the ear canal known as otitis externa (inflammation of the external part of the ear). The ear canal is red and swollen and appropriate treatment with a combination of antibiotics and steroids is usually curative. In these two cases, however, the appearance was normal and the distribution of the itchy/burning sensation suggested once again that the culprit must be either some form of allergy or a disturbance of the sensory nerves to the ear, or malocclusion of the jaw.

Allergy

♦ 'I suggest she should stop using hairsprays. If that does not work she should change her shampoo. Should hairspray be essential to her happiness and good grooming, then wash the ears, face and neck directly after spraying the hair.'

♦ 'Regarding the itchy ear problem, I too had this and found it was due to the spongy covers on earphones.'

♦ 'The ants in the ear syndrome can be cleared up with the simple expedient of keeping as much of the ear as possible from water and not letting a drop inside.'

♦ 'I have the "ants and spiders", a patch about saucer size centred on my left ear, half in and half out of the hairline. The sensation is just as though a few small insects are crawling over the skin – you can feel the hairs parting to let them through. I mentioned it to my brother-in-law who suffers similarly. He has seen doctors and specialists to no avail, but his wife suggested Vaseline Hand and Nail Formula and it worked for him. For me, one generous application and it was totally clear. It did return a few weeks later and again I treated it and it just stopped.'

Nerve Root Pressure

♦ 'The sides of the face are supplied by nerves from the cervical vertebrae and pressure on that nerve's root can sometimes give rise to such symptoms. I recently had a patient whose symptoms cleared completely after one session of manipulation at the level of the first and second cervical vertebrae.'

Malocclusion of the Jaw

'Many years ago I had had a back tooth removed and for a long time afterwards I found it difficult to find a comfortable position for my jaw. My upper and lower jaws did not seem to fit together as they used to and it caused me a lot of discomfort. It seemed to me then that the misalignment was due to the removal of that tooth and over the years it has gradually become worse. This finally led to my peculiar problem of itchy ears. While it is still not cured I have learned to control it. When the itching starts I open my mouth slightly and "wiggle" my jaws. After a minute or two the itching stops and I never now get the unbearable burning itch which so spoiled my life before.'

SORE EARS

Query 75-year-old Miss P.C. from Surrey writes: 'For about the last ten years I have woken frequently when lying on either side suffering from very sore ears. *The soreness affects the line of rigid muscle which runs alongside the soft outer rim of the ear down to the lobe.* Two doctors and a plastic surgeon have told me they had not encountered this before and there is nothing to be done. This is distressing!'

Comment Soreness of the outer ear can be due to one or other of the following two syndromes.

Restricted Blood Supply

♦ 'I suggest this lady's problem is due to a restricted blood supply to the fleshy part of the ear. This restriction could arise because of the weight of her head on a too-firm pillow, therefore obstructing the flow of blood to the part.'

The precipitating factor appears to be that the ear 'folds over' when asleep as described by two readers:

♦ 'On inspection I have noticed my left ear has a larger flap at the top whereas my right ear lies quite flat close to the ear and I suspect that the left ear's larger flap tends to double over when I sleep on that side.'
♦ 'My right ear is thinner, more flexible and sticks out more than the left and I have always thought this problem is caused by sleeping with the ear curled over. Possibly the squashing affects the circulation and the pain sets in when the head is moved again and circulation begins to return to normal.'

Remedies The appropriate remedy, obviously enough, is somehow to reduce the pressure on the ear by one of a variety of ways:

♦ 'I now sleep on my back – which incidentally I find very comfortable and only occasionally have the pain and soreness along the side of my ear.'

♦ 'My own solution is to cup my hand over the ear, thus keeping the pressure off and I hope I do it automatically as I turn from side to side during sleep.'

♦ 'The answer is to change to a very soft pillow. Unless I sleep on the best quality goosedown pillow I have a miserable night. When I used to travel a lot I took my own pillow with me because hotels have a nasty habit of providing pillows with manmade fibre stuffing, absolute torture!'

♦ 'I have found using two pillows helpful. The top pillow should be smaller and firmer and made of foam or similar material. Place it further back so it just supports the head and the ear can nestle with no pressure on the lower pillow.'

Chondrodermatitis Helicis Chronica

This impressive sounding diagnosis, as so often, is merely the description in Latin of what appears to be the matter – chronic inflammation of the skin overlying the helical cartilage of the outer ear. The pain is centred on red, oval-shaped nodules with raised rolled edges which often contains a crust or scale.

Treatment

♦ 'I have had the same problem over the years and have obtained relief by treating the sores with zinc and castor oil ointment – the same treatment we used for the sore bottoms of our babies. The sores heal in a few days and the cure lasts for quite a time.'

♦ 'Injection of steroid directly into the nodule, which produces resolution of the lesion within two to three weeks in about 50 per cent of cases.'

♦ 'My surgeon performed a small operation to correct what he termed "an area of damaged cartilage which became inflamed". There is nothing to the operation really and I am glad to say I have suffered no pain since.'

YELLOW EARS

This is an unresolved mystery, described by Mrs M.B. from Seaford:

> I have never had any major illnesses or skin complaints but for the last few months I have suffered from intense itching of the neck, limbs and torso together with a yellow discoloration of the top half of both ear lobes. The specialist has been very concerned and painstaking and I have had numerous blood tests all of which were negative and a skin biopsy. My specialist took me before a panel of consultants none of whom could find any reason for the itching or the yellow ears. Steroid tablets can control the itching and allow the rash to clear but I suffer side-effects with them.

The Nose

The nose is a wonderful thing, combining the three separate functions of contributing to the aesthetic beauty of its owner, acting as the organ of smell and moisturizing and filtering the air before it enters the lungs. In fulfilling this latter role, the lining of the nose comes into contact with viruses, bacteria and irritants which in turn are responsible for the common cold and allergic rhinitis (inflammation of the lining of the nose) respectively, with their symptoms of nasal congestion, nasal discharge and sneezing.

The two main forms of allergic rhinitis are 'seasonal' – limited to a few months a year induced by pollen and other allergens and associated with the usual hay fever symptoms; then there is perennial (or continuous) rhinitis where exposure to the allergens – which may or may not be known – continue throughout the year. Treatment is quite straightforward and involves avoiding – where possible – the allergens, steam inhalation and a steroid nasal spray.

There are, however, several more unusual variants of these nasal problems.

RUNNY NOSE

Query 1 Mr J.D. from Cumbria writes:

> *I have suffered from running nose and watering eyes for many years* and it gets worse as time goes by. My favourite pastimes are golf and fell walking and I had hoped to enjoy both in my retirement. However, a constantly dripping nose and streaming eyes are depriving me of much of my hoped-for pleasure. I can soak five or six large handkerchiefs during a round of golf and the beautiful countryside which surrounds me on my walks is diffused by almost constant tears.

Query 2 Mrs N.S. from Crewe writes: 'As soon as I rise in the morning *my nose starts "dripping" just like a leaking tap which needs a new washer*. It stops for two or three hours to resume again most evenings. It is extremely embarrassing particularly when shopping and having to cope with a purse, purchases, change, etc.'

Comment This is an exaggerated form of 'allergic' rhinitis, for which the following suggestions were made:

Identify and avoid the cause

- *Coffee*: 'I have endured dripping nose syndrome for years. During that time I have drunk about eight cups of strong coffee daily. Recently I gave it up and felt dreadful for three days and nights but the end result is that I feel younger, more energetic, less tired and – no dripping nose.'
- *House dust mite*: 'The cause may be an allergic reaction to the house dust mite. I too used to suffer similarly until I had my first attack of asthma. I followed the usual advice about buying a foam pillow and keeping it clean by washing it every three months, vacuuming my bedclothes, etc. I have not only been clear of any further asthma attacks, but my nose has also "dried up" too.'

♦ *Spectacles*: 'Some years ago when I was discussing runny noses with a friend in a pub, she said she had suffered from one ever since she started wearing glasses. She said she had heard the runny nose was caused by the glasses aggravating a nerve in the bridge of the nose. Now I wear glasses all the time and when I get up in the morning and replace my specs, the tap opens for some 30 or 40 minutes. Thereafter I only have to blow or wipe my nose once or twice every hour. Remove the glasses and the problem stops immediately.

Medication

♦ Tony Narula, ENT surgeon from Leicester Royal Infirmary, advises that in the older age group, a runny nose is often due to an imbalance of the action of the autonomic nerves in the nose. Steroid sprays are therefore ineffective but ipatroprium bromide which blocks the neurotransmitter chemicals 'turns off the tap', and may need to be complemented with the antihistamine spray Azelastine.

♦ The anti-asthma spray Ventolin taken as two puffs a minute can 'stop the flow of watery mucus'. 'I have adopted this procedure with great success and only occasionally do I need to repeat it later in the day.'

♦ I am afflicted in the same way but thankfully I have discovered that a dose of the homeopathic remedy Natrumur stops the dripping nose almost instantly.

Exclude other causes When the runny nose is profuse and persistent and limited to one nostril, the rare but important possibility of a leak of cerebro spinal fluid (CFS) from around the brain must be considered as illustrated in the following case history.

Three months previously a 21-year-old man had an acute onset of rhinorrhoea (runny nose) not associated with nasal block or allergy. Treatments with antihistamines and steroid sprays had failed to alleviate the symptoms. Examination revealed a normal nose. When the patient bent forward there was a copious flow of clear fluid from the right nostril. The fluid was collected and confirmed to be CSF. Two months later an exploratory operation revealed a small defect at the base of the skull which was repaired. He made a good recovery and eight months later was free of symptoms.

DRY NOSE

Query Mr G.C. from Dorset writes: 'I suffer from a *dry irritating nose*. From time to time it can be quite sore but most often just plain uncomfortable. I have seen an ENT consultant who could not account for my condition. I have tried various personal treatments of vaseline, sprays, saline washouts and creams to no effect. The right nostril is the main offender.'

Comment The sensation of dry irritation reflects the important role of the fluid secreted by the lining of the nose in moisturizing inhaled air as it is drawn into the lungs. The dryness may follow an acute upper respiratory tract infection, be a side-effect of drugs such as isotretinoin for acne and doxasosin for raised blood pressure, or may be part of a more generalized drying up of the mucus membranes known as the sicca (dry) syndrome most commonly associated with Sjogren's syndrome, so named after the Swedish ophthalmologist who first described it. Central heating and gas fires are exacerbating factors. Several readers commented that mystified doctors tend to resort to empirical treatments with anti-allergy nasal sprays such as Rhinocort or Beconase. These, however, can be counterproductive, exacerbating the sensation of dryness and not infrequently causing bleeding from the nostrils.

The following measures were suggested.

General measures

♦ *Vaseline*: Dr J.M. Campbell of Bromley writes: Vaseline should be regularly applied at night (using a cotton bud) and several times during the day if necessary. This helps the nasal lining to retain more moisture. Should bleeding occur then cod liver oil should be applied once or twice followed by a return to the vaseline. Persevere with the treatment. Adequate fluid intake is essential. Alternatives to vaseline are Sudocrem and Savlon.

♦ *Nasal irrigation*: Dr J. Nuutinen from Finland writes: Nasal irrigation with saline has been used since the beginning of the century to remove crusts and improve nasal breathing. The solution is commercially available (Humidose) in a bottle equipped with a metred dose pump giving 0.09ml of solution at each spray.

♦ *Sjogren's syndrome*: Those with Sjogren's syndrome will have to combine the above remedies with additional treatments for dry eye and dry mouth. 'I use Hypromellose eyedrops during the day and sweet almond oil helps me through the night. I also make my own moisturisers with glycerine, oil and peppermint.'

THROBBING NOSTRIL

Query Mrs J. from Cumbria writes: 'I lose a lot of sleep because when *I lie down at night I start to get a very painful throbbing up my right nostril*. If I manage to get to sleep I am later awakened by intense pain. There is some relief if I lie on my left side, but I can't sleep comfortably in that position.'

Comment The only suggestion was that this might be due to a deviated nasal septum.

> May I respectfully suggest that this is due to a deviated septum. I used the nasal decongenstant Otrivine which at the time gave almost instant relief, but was told to stop it as it was more of a long-term aggravant. Relief is also obtained by lying on the other side to clear the blockage together with a hot water compress applied to the bridge of the nose, e.g. a flannel soaked in very hot water. I eventually had a corrective operation and the problem disappeared.

EXCESS MUCUS/CATARRH

Query 1 Miss C.C. from Suffolk writes: 'For the past four years I have had *excess mucus draining down the back of my throat* that wakes me several times a night and I often feel sick on waking from swallowing it. It also settles on my chest causing discomfort.'

Query 2 Mr M.R. from Essex writes:

> Five years ago I developed what I thought was the familiar beginning of a cold: instead it disappeared after a day or two, leaving me with what I took to be catarrh accompanied each morning by *a sore throat, a dry mouth and a persistently wet nose. My upper throat has remained excessively sensitive* ever since and all too frequently while eating causing me to cough violently followed immediately by equally violent sneezes. Catarrh persists, as does the morning sore throat and nose dampness.

Comment Excess nasal mucus is a most distressing symptom which may arise from the nasal lining itself or the sinuses and which, particularly at night, drips down the back of the throat into the lungs to cause a distressing cough. It may be associated with allergic or perennial rhinitis when appropriate medication is indicated, or may be part of the runny nose (rhinorrhea) syndrome already mentioned. Antibiotics may be appropriate if there is evidence of bacterial infection. Specific suggestions include the following.

(i) *Decongestant*: Several readers reported a good response to the standard decongestant medications – such as Sudafed and Visclair – which doctors may be reluctant to recommend under the impression that they are not very effective.

(ii) *Salt water*: An ENT consultant who himself suffers from excess catarrh recommends the following salt water remedy which he uses twice a day: 'Pour a little salt into the bowl of a tablespoon containing warm water and with head held back, sniff the liquid up the nostril. It has worked miracles for me, and others. The mucus is released immediately.'

(iii) *Garlic oil capsules*: 'I take one 1000mg capsule of garlic oil before going to bed and find I wake up with a clear throat. If I forget to take the capsule or forget to renew the supply in the bathroom cabinet, the problem returns.'

(iv) *Food sensitivity*: There is no doubt that certain foods can predispose to formation of catarrh: the main culprit being dairy products. A reader reports how her daughter inadvertently discovered that milk was a causative factor:

> My daughter suffered from sinus problems and excess catarrh badly in her teens and early 20s, needing or rather being prescribed, a variety of drugs that did little for her and some which made her worse. When she decided to leave home and have a flat of her own she was very short of cash. In an effort to cut every bill she could, she opted to have skimmed milk instead of whole milk, which was dearer. She got through the winter with no sinusitis or any related problem. Better finances meant she went back to whole milk and back came the sinus problem. Back on skimmed milk and the problem disappeared. So change of milk meant lower milk bills, no prescription charges, no wasting doctors' time and relief for her. Perhaps it will work for others.

Humans, it would seem, are not the only ones who are sensitive to dairy products in this way, as Dr Layinka Swinburne reports in the Lancet:

> The patient, aged 15, had had a cough for at least five years and a constantly running nose with a discharge of thick mucus. Her voice became hoarse and very often she could only mouth her messages silently. Many therapies were tried including antibiotics, both in short courses and longer lower dose regimes. Over the past year no treatment has had much effect. I realized that if she had two legs instead of four I would be considering a diagnosis of milk allergy. We stopped her daily treat of a saucer of cream at coffee time which she had learnt to demand in a special voice. After 48 hours her nose dried up, the cough stopped completely, and she could purr without bringing on a bout of coughing.

A further, if more unlikely, culprit is orange juice:

> Some time ago I used to suffer from very severe nasal congestion. I tried all sorts of tablets but they only gave temporary relief. Then by chance I had to go away on a course for about a week, and lo and behold the congestion cleared up. I sat down and had a think about what I had eaten or drunk at this hotel and how it differed from what I normally have at home. By a process of elimination it turned out, to my utter astonishment, to be orange juice. Even an eggcup full would set it off. It came as a bit of a blow as I was very fond of orange. The cure was instantaneous.

SNEEZING

Sneezing is a highly efficient means of dislodging particles from the nose, which occurs in two distinct phases. In the first, the lining of the nose responds to some irritating particle by becoming engorged and secretes a clear mucus substance in which it will be expelled. The nasal engorgement, in turn, stimulates a series of deep rapid inspirations, storing a large volume of air within the chest. The second phase starts once the pressure in the lungs has passed a critical point. The combination of elastic recoil of lung tissue and the interaction of muscle of the chest and abdominal wall, hurtles air back out of the lungs at a speed of 100 ft per second, expelling the mucus droplets in a fine mist to a distance of around six feet.

The common causes of sneezing are a viral infection or some pollutant in the air or, for hay fever sufferers, pollen – but for some, especially when the sneezing is repetitive and explosive, the explanation may be less obvious.

Query 1 Dr G.T. from Northants writes on behalf of a 64-year-old accountant friend who has always enjoyed good health, but for 30 years been subject to *bouts of unprovoked evening sneezing*: 'These occur on average five times every week and can be quite alarming to those who do not know him. He usually sneezes nine times in rapid succession *with no forewarning, no nasal irritation and little mucus; there is no eye watering or deafness*. Even more curiously the attack almost invariably occurs within a few minutes of 9 p.m. – and when he is abroad his nose sets itself to the new time zone within 24 hours!'

Query 2 Mr G.H. from the Wirral writes:

The sneezing fits happen more often than not in the early morning and are frequently a daily occurrence, although I will sometimes go for a week without one. *I sneeze violently between six and 12 times over a period of a couple of minutes.* Interestingly, my late father also suffered from sneezing fits – his were far more severe often lasting for over ten minutes and leaving him like a wet rag.

My brother has similar fits, as do my two sons and also my two nephews.

Comment Both sudden changes of temperature ('If I get into the car which has been outside all night, in a few seconds I'll be off') and looking into bright lights or sunlight ('which can be hazardous on motorways') can precipitate sneezing but there are some other less obvious sources:

♦ *Aspirin*: Many people nowadays regularly take a small dose of aspirin to protect against a heart attack or stroke. This, or other similar types of non-steroidal anti-inflammatory drugs, can precipitate daily episodic attacks described by one reader as 'an itchy tickling in the throat, followed by convulsive coughing, often ending in about six almighty sneezes'.

♦ *Sugar*: 'At the age of 18, I began my first employment as an assistant in the laboratory of a factory where confectionery of numerous kinds was made. Several years passed and I began to experience attacks of sneezing, which became more violent as time passed. I could saturate a handkerchief in a matter of minutes. On one occasion I came upon an article in an American journal by a dentist who claimed that ingestion of considerable quantities of sugar could cause symptoms exactly as I was experiencing. From that time I reduced as far as my duties allowed my consumption of confectionery. At home I was careful as far as possible to avoid iced cakes. To my great relief, my symptoms quickly disappeared.

♦ *Cheap white wine*: 'I have uncontrolled sneezing and runny nose within one to two hours of drinking a half bottle of cheap white wine – which usually has a very high content of sulphur dioxide.'

♦ *Newspaper print*: 'I often wondered why I sneezed early mornings at 7.30 a.m. then again at lunch time and sometimes at 5.00 p.m. I then realized after some time that these are the times I open a fresh newspaper and there is some suggestion I am allergic to the printers' ink, which is not always very dry.'

Treatment Standard anti-allergy medication with antihistamines and steroid nasal sprays are of value. Other suggestions include:

(i) *Pressure*: Pressing on my upper lip immediately below my nose sometimes alleviates the fit.
(ii) *Nose blowing*: After sneezing, one should immediately blow one's nose. Repetitive sneezing becomes a habit which is broken by blowing the nose.
(iii) *Chocolate*: Whenever a friend took me out for dinner he would, at the end of the meal, always start to sneeze and sneeze and sneeze. No reason, no cheese course, no coffee, no time for these things, because as soon as the main course was finished the sneezing would start. On one occasion he had some chocolate and the sneezing stopped instantly. Now he does not go into a restaurant without at least the facility to obtain an 'After Eight' chocolate mint.

The Mouth

The mouth is much the most sensitive and sensuous part of the body, through whose various attributes – lips, teeth, gums, tongue and palate – sensations of taste, mastication and physical contact are mediated. For the most part, gratefully, mouth ailments are readily recognizable and correctable by the relevant specialist, whether dentist, dermatologist, maxillo facial surgeon, and so on. But for the mystery syndromes described here, the mouth appears entirely normal and the explanation elusive.

BURNING MOUTH SYNDROME

Query Miss M.L. from Somerset writes: 'I have been *troubled with a sore mouth, and burning itching lips* for the past four months and am getting desperate. I have consulted both my doctor and dentist, knowledgeable and experienced men, and tried all the usual treatments – antifungal treatment, mouthwashes, zinc supplement – but to no avail.'

Comment This problem is known as Burning Mouth Syndrome (BMS), of which three types are recognized:

♦ Type 1 – Burning is not present on waking, but worsens throughout the day.
♦ Type 2 – Burning is present from the minute the patient wakes in the morning until they go to bed.
♦ Type 3 – Burning is experienced on some days only and tends to affect unusual sites such as the floor of the mouth or throat.

BMS is an abnormality of the sensory nerves within the mouth and so, by definition, its appearance will be normal. Several possible precipitating factors have, however, been identified:

♦ *Toothpaste*: A lady dentist from Cambridge and long-time sufferer from BMS found, if perhaps paradoxically, toothpaste to be the culprit: 'A soft toothbrush, children's toothpaste and less zealous though sufficient brushing' improved her symptoms.

The responsible chemical is propyl nicotinate, which is incorporated into several toothpastes in order to improve the microcirculation of the blood. Sorbic acid used as a preservative in foods as well as in ointments and creams has also been incriminated.

♦ *Dental work*: The use of local anaesthetic injections to numb the pain during dental work may give rise to BMS because of the presence of the chemical sodium metabisulfite. The same salt is also widely used as a preservative in wine, beer and fruit juice and vegetables such as potatoes, and some other drugs including antibiotics and steroids.

♦ *Miscellaneous*: Other precipitants of BMS were reported by readers, including culpeppers, glasses washed in the dishwasher, spray perfumes, prescription eyedrops, air fresheners, tomatoes, the sweetener Aspartame and nail varnish.

♦ *Thrush*: Dr Winson Huang from the University of Connecticut writes: 'Candidiasis (oral thrush) has been reported to be a causative factor in BMS. Its presence in the mouth is increased and there are reports of remission after oral antifungal treatment.'

♦ *Acid reflux*: 'The nocturnal regurgitation of acidic fluids' was identified as the cause of BMS by one reader who obtained relief by using 'an extra pillow at night' and taking the acid-suppressant drug Losec. Dr Mario Garcia-Bravatti from Guatemala describes the case of a 35-year-old woman with both BMS and symptoms of heartburn. 'During three weeks treatment with the acid suppressant Losec she improved progressively, with her pain disappearing entirely within a month. She then stopped therapy and her symptoms promptly returned.'

Treatment When no precipitant is identified, there is no alternative other than to treat the condition with one or other of a variety of empirical remedies.

(i) *Mouthwash*: One teaspoon of equal parts of elixir of Benadryl and Kaolin and pectate retained in the mouth for one to two minutes and then spat out, 20 to 30 minutes before meals is reported as being 'helpful'. Cold apple juice as a mouthwash may be similarly effective.

(ii) *Drug treatment*: Various drugs used primarily in the treatment of depression can help some patients. These include amitryptiline and clonazepam. The form of psychotherapy known as cognitive therapy has also been used.

SORE TONGUE

Query 1 84-year-old Mr W.M. from Cornwall writes:

My tongue has been *very sore for the last 20 months, having a permanently 'scalded' feeling*. I eat a balanced diet and drink nothing to excess. My doctor, dentist and pharmacist at the local chemist can all only recommend vitamin B complex, which I have been taking for the past year. It appeared to help for a little while but now has little effect.

Query 2 52-year-old Mrs D.M. from Devon writes: 'For the last year I have suffered *a very sore tip and side of my tongue* *and sore lower lip*. There is hardly anything to see. Medical and alternative remedies have not helped. What a relief it would be to eat and talk again in comfort.'

Comment There are two recognized medical conditions that can give rise to a sensation of a sore tongue: pernicious anaemia (due to vitamin B12 deficiency) and lichen planus (a skin disorder which may respond to steroids). The general view, however, is these complaints of sore tongue are a variant of Burning Mouth Syndrome which may, in certain cases, similarly be induced by sensitivity to food or chemicals.

♦ *Benzoate preservatives*: 'For several years I suffered intermittently from a tongue which was either sore at the tip and edges or felt "scalded". Patch tests showed I was allergic, among other things, to a group of chemicals (benzoates) which are widely used as food preservatives. "Sore tongue" sufferers can start to help themselves by avoiding processed food and drink as much as possible, particularly those items which are kept after opening for any length of time – such as salad creams and fruit squashes. After meals, rinse the mouth well and brush the tongue gently but do not use coloured toothpastes. Read the small print on packaging and avoid E numbers 210–219 inclusive. My tongue is now comfortable most of the time, but occasionally the problem recurs if I have made an unwise choice when eating out.'

♦ *Toothpaste*: 'I too have had this problem, which was caused by using Armand and Hammer toothpaste with baking soda which was so widely and convincingly advertised some time ago. It was extremely painful and worrying, but cleared up within a couple of days on going back to dear old Macleans!'

♦ *Amalgam*: 'My wife, following a visit to her dentist, developed a soreness on the side of her tongue which was first thought to be due to roughness of a new amalgam filling on the side of her tooth. Despite polishing the filling there was no improvement. Eventually after several visits to her doctor it was concluded that it was an allergic reaction to the amalgam filling. The dentist recommended crowning the tooth which, while costly, cleared up the soreness.'

♦ *Lipstick*: 'I have recently suffered from a burning tongue along with my lips. I wondered if it could possibly be an allergic reaction to a lipstick. I duly stopped the one I suspected and I am no longer suffering.'

Treatment The treatment for sore tongue runs along similar lines to BMS. There are reports of benefit from vitamin B6 and a reader advises the following coping strategies:

(i) Think of it always as a 'tingling' rather than a burning sensation.
(ii) Think of something else, read a book or even better, write one.
(iii) Hot foods, curries, chilli and ginger mask it. Sips of cold milk are soothing.

GEOGRAPHIC TONGUE

Query Mrs A.L. from London writes:

For six months *the tips and sides of my tongue were very sore, as was the inside of my mouth. Some foods made the mouth more painful.* All fruits, including melon and banana, were out and the only meal I could eat painlessly was porridge! I was referred to an oral surgeon who diagnosed the condition as 'geographic' tongue.

Comment Geographic tongue is so called because its main feature is its unusual appearance, where swollen red patches move around the surface of the tongue resembling, as it were, continents on the surface of the globe. The main symptom is a burning pain when consuming highly seasoned spicy foods, fruits, tomatoes and alcohol. Treatment is not very satisfactory, but covering the tongue with gentian violet or applying the vitamin A derivative tretinoin have been reported to be beneficial.

BLACK HAIRY TONGUE

Black hairy tongue, as its name implies, is a condition where *the back of the tongue is covered with an abnormal coating of black 'hairs'* which can tickle the back of the throat. Dr J.A. Langtry describes a case and the appropriate treatment:

> A 72-year-old woman presented with a six-month history of black hairy tongue following a course of antibiotics for cystitis. The posterior half of the tongue was black and velvety in appearance. There was no improvement during treatment with antifungal medication. After one month of daily treatment with topical tretinoin gel and brushing with a soft toothbrush clearing was achieved. There has been no recurrence in the two years since treatment.

SWOLLEN LIPS

Query 1 Mrs P.M., a 65-year-old former general nurse from Hampshire, writes:

> Every few weeks *I get a swelling on either my top or lower lip on the right side* and as I write this my top lip resembles the 'hanging lip of Babylon'. I showed the swelling to a couple of doctors when I worked as a nurse who had no idea what might have caused it. One suggested antihistamines, the other offered to biff me on the left side to even things up. The swelling usually occurs at night but I can actually feel it coming up, like the starting of a cold sore. It begins to go down after a few hours and is virtually gone by the next day.

Query 2 Mrs P.G. from Exeter writes:

> *I would wake in the morning with a large and very embarrassing swelling on my face, generally on the bottom half,* especially near the mouth and nose. My main memory of the problem was total embarrassment as my face was almost unrecognizable and I was at an age when such problems mattered more than perhaps they would now!

Comment This is a variant of the allergic condition known as angioneurotic oedema – a misleading term as the term 'angioneurotic' conveys the impression this may be a neurotic disorder. This is not the case, rather the origin of the term reflects the original concept of the condition where the nerves (neuro) influence the blood vessels (angio) to cause an outpouring of fluid from the blood vessels into the surrounding tissue, to cause swelling (oedema).

There is a strong association with the itchy blotches of urticaria and it is usually induced by an allergic reaction.

- ♦ *Pears*: 'I had similar symptoms and noticed it happened after eating pears. My gums were also quite sore. I then tried removing the skins and found I could eat the pears with no ill effect.'
- ♦ *Toothpaste*: When toothpaste reaches the outer lip during teeth cleaning, it can cause the lips to swell and become tender.
- ♦ *Washing powder*: The fact that she suffers swelling on her lips at night suggests it might be to do with the washing powder or fabric conditioner which she uses to wash her bed linen.
- ♦ *Food allergy*: 'Years ago I had the same problem, which proved to be sudden food allergy – in my case to fish – which living near the sea, I had eaten for years with no adverse reaction. Four to six hours after my evening meal, my top lip would swell up and subside over the next four hours. Then after several weeks and the onset of the next attack, the other side would also swell so the whole top lip became affected. It is possible more than one allergen is involved. A distinct possibility is salicylate acid found mainly in aspirin, tomatoes, strawberries and raspberries, also possibly wheat.'
- ♦ *Drugs*: The swollen lips may be a side-effect of drugs, of which the most important are the ace inhibitors used in the treatment of hypertension.

Treatment

(i) *Antihistamines*: Antihistamine pills can stop an attack, though if taken in the morning, the lip and face are already swollen.

(ii) *Ice cubes*: 'My last attack was nearly one year ago when my lip burned and swelled I immediately applied an ice pack – and miraculously it promptly subsided. Is it eureka?'

(iii) *Tranexamic acid*: Dr R.A. Thompson from Birmingham describes the case of a 24-year-old married woman who had 'intermittent attacks of angioneurotic oedema for about five years, occurring almost every day. She was given a trial of Tranexamic acid, 1g three times a day and the effect was dramatic. The attacks ceased completely, the dose was gradually reduced and she has remained symptom free for three months.'

MOUTH BLISTERS

Query Mr D.A.T., a 76-year-old company director from Bucks, writes:

> I suffer from *massive blood blisters on my tongue* caused by simple things such as a rough edge on an apple, biscuits, toast etc. even when eating with great care, as I am, of course, prone to do. None of the medications I have tried have helped to prevent the blisters or harden the tongue to prevent them happening.

Comment This is a rare, chronic blistering disease known as Benign Mucosal Penphigoid, which affects the mucous membrane of the mouth and genital tract. It can be a very frightening experience, as another reader comments:

> The last really bad happening occurred whilst eating in a restaurant. A tiny fragment of red pepper was the cause. It produced a tiny graze which instantly erupted into a blood blister so huge that it filled my mouth and I thought I would choke. I raced to the loo and frantically tried to 'pop' it which I did in part, and all the while spitting clot after clot of the brightest red blood. I lost a lot and went back to the table as white as a sheet.'

Well-recognized precipitants include hot drinks, while ginger biscuits – 'virtually a guarantee of a blood blister'.

Treatment Treatment is described as 'difficult'. Mr B.S. Crawford, a surgeon from Sheffield, writes:

Rough dentistry and obvious dietary causes should be avoided. Some people carry a needle with which to puncture a blister before it enlarges. The larger the blister, the larger and more painful the ulcer. Before a meal a cold drink may help, reinforced by sips during eating. Anything like ice cream or yoghurt afterwards may help. The mouth spray Eludil is also recommended. 'It eases the pain almost instantly and clears the blisters in about three days'.

DROOLING

Query Mrs M.S., a 73-year-old retired librarian from Yorkshire, writes:

I always thought it was only senile people who dribbled but although I am in perfect health, there is something that I have endured for several months now and I find it very upsetting. *Nothing specific seems to cause it but there is a constant trickle of saliva from the (mainly right hand) side of my mouth* and I can feel drops forming on my chin. Mopping this up constantly is beginning to mark my skin which is becoming red and scaly.

Comment Drooling is a well-recognized symptom in Parkinson's disease (due to a reduced ability to swallow saliva) and in children with cerebral palsy and other forms of developmental disorder. It would seem to be very unusual for it to occur as a solitary symptom in someone who is otherwise well, but it might be reasonable to investigate the treatments for the above conditions in the hope that they might perhaps be of benefit.

Treatment

(i) *Parkinson's disease*: It would seem sensible to consider the possibility of early Parkinson's and initiate a course of treatment to see whether or not it is of benefit.

(ii) *Medical treatment to reduce salivary flow*: The drug benzhexol acts on the nerves that control the action of the salivary glands to reduce their flow.

(iii) *Surgical reduction of salivary flow*: Mr B.K. Young of the Royal Brisbane Hospital writes: 'Surgery is indicated for marked or severe cases of drooling but any method must still allow sufficient volume of flow for mastication and oral hygiene.' He recommends an operation involving redirection of the flow from the parotid gland into the back of the pharynx, which may be combined with the removal of both salivary glands under the jaw.

TEETH GRINDING

Query 1 'My 84-year-old mother continually *grinds her teeth* and, when not doing that, keeps on moving her lower jaw from side to side. She finds this very distressing and says people do not seem to be able to avoid constantly mentioning it.'

Query 2 Mrs S.J. from Sussex writes: 'I too move my lower jaw from side to side, which is an involuntary habit and most embarrassing. I can keep my jaw still, but it is a great effort and I have to concentrate like mad.

Comment This teeth grinding has a name – oral dyskinesia (literally 'abormal movement of the mouth') and is due to an abnormality of the nerves that control the movement of the mouth. It is not unusual in the older age group, affecting approximately one in five. The following two precipitating or exacerbating factors should be considered:

◆ *Side-effects of drugs*: Teeth grinding is a common side-effect of several different types of medication, including those for epilepsy, Parkinson's and psychological problems (antidepressants and benzodiazepines).
◆ *Poorly fitting dentures*: Dr Howard Suture of the University of Illinois describes four patients with severe oral dyskinesia which was found to be due to poorly fitting dentures. 'A 49-year-old white man with a normal medical history who had complete dentures for many years, gradually developed symptoms of oral dyskinesia over a period of eight months. Muscle relaxants, tranquillizers and a job change did not help. Following replacement with a new set of complete dentures, all symptoms of oral

dyskinesia are now essentially eliminated. Removal of the dentures induces almost complete relapse within twenty-four hours.'

♦ *Clonazepam*: There is a report of 'noticeable improvement' in two people with oral dyskinesia following treatment with the drug Clonazepam.

PAINFUL GUMS

Query A 64-year-old former hairdresser, Mrs S.B. from Yorkshire:

The gums and teeth of mainly the right side of the top of my mouth are swollen and very painful. When very bad I feel very dizzy and tired, but at night when lying down the pain is less. Two oral surgeons are stumped and physiotherapy and exercise for the neck muscles have not helped.

Comment There are many reasons for gum pain, from infection (gingivitis) to tooth abscess, and these can usually be sorted out by a dentist or a gum specialist known as a periodontologist. Two suggestions for this lady's problem are as follows:

♦ *Herpes infection*: 'Two years ago I started having painful gums and teeth just on one side (left) and this coincides with a recurrence of the herpes virus, which starts in my head and then works its way down affecting my ear, the inside of my nose, and then my mouth and neck. The gums become pink, sensitive and very painful and my teeth feel as if I have the sort of toothache that should take me to the dentist. Pain in all these areas goes off after a couple of days, leaving me quite ragged.'

♦ *HRT*: The oestrogen component of HRT and the Pill and the high oestrogen levels during pregnancy can, it is claimed, cause painful and bleeding gums. The only treatment recommended by readers is from a lady from Surrey: 'After months of pain and after trying various remedies to no avail I was told by a top oral consultant to try massaging sensodyne toothpaste into my gums. It gave me almost instant relief. My sister has the same problem and it worked for her too.'

PAINFUL TEETH

Toothache is bad enough, but thanks to the dental profession there is usually little difficulty in having it sorted out. Sometimes, however, dental treatment is of no help, which raises the possibility that the source of the pain must lie elsewhere. Here there are two possible diagnoses.

Neuralgia

Persistent pain may be a variant of the facial pain syndromes (see Facial Pain) as described in the following case history by Dr Lewis Reik from Connecticut:

> A 38-year-old woman had had toothache and facial pain for three years. *At first the throbbing pain was centred in the right lower first molar and second pre-molar and occurred episodically at intervals for several days*, each attack lasting for 12–24 hours. Although the X-rays were normal, her teeth were extracted. It gradually became continuous, steadily gripping with a superimposed throbbing component. She became depressed and was treated with a wide variety of drugs including anti-inflammatories and anti-anxiety drugs, to no avail. On examination there was spasm and tenderness of both jaw joints (TMJs) and spasm and tenderness of the left masseter muscle. The depression was treated with trazodone but left the pain unaffected. Addition of methysergide, 4mg daily, eliminated the pain.

Phantom Tooth Pain

Dr I. Marbach writes:

> *Phantom tooth pain* (PTP) resembles other phantom pain syndromes that arise after amputation and injury. Sufferers also complain of toothache in previously extracted teeth – a classic phantom sensation. *The pain is described as a constant, dull, deep ache with occasional spontaneous sharp exacerbations.* Many report a brief symptom-free period on awakening. This lasts from

seconds to minutes. Otherwise the pain is constant. Usually the onset of PTP follows dental or surgical procedures such as root canal treatment or tooth extraction.

He advises a step-wise method for treatment:

Step 1: Reassure the patient that pain can occur even when the structure (tooth, nerve) is removed.

Step 2: Put the patient on Gabapentin, starting at 100mg. Give it sufficient time (one month) and increase the dose before trying other drugs.

Step 3: Consider nerve block therapy with local anaesthetic and steroids. Avoid dental and surgical procedures.

3
The Senses: Vision, Hearing, Taste and Smell

The four senses of hearing, sight, taste and smell are staggeringly sensitive and vulnerable to a host of differing misfortunes, all of which have specific symptoms that will require the attention of the relevant specialists. The following are of interest as being unusual, puzzling or difficult to treat.

Vision

HALLUCINATIONS

Query Mrs A.R., a retired nurse from Wiltshire writes:

> I visit a delightful mentally alert 85-year-old lady who lives alone and whose eyesight is deteriorating. Some weeks *she sees on her living room walls the most vivid 'pictures'*: humans, objects, flowers, a woman with a flowing skirt walking down a staircase, and many more. These images last a few seconds then fade. She describes them all so vividly when I am with her that I feel quite deprived: instead of these fascinating moving pictures all I see is a blank wall! My friend is anxious to hear if other people share this private film show.

Comment Hallucinations are part of the same spectrum as dreaming, it is just that they occur while awake rather than asleep. They often go unrecognized by doctors as those experiencing them may not reveal the symptoms for fear of being labelled as 'mad'. Virtually any form of brain disturbance can result in visual hallucinations – drugs, neurological disease, psychiatric conditions – but the concern here is their occurrence in those who are otherwise quite normal except for having very poor vision. These are sometimes called 'release hallucinations', because they are released from within the brain in response to the absence of normal visual input from the external world. The philosopher Charles Bonnet first described them in 1760 in his grandfather, who had had cataract surgery and at the age of 89 began to see brightly coloured and organized visions. Two further case reports are as follows:

> A 64-year-old man whose eyesight has deteriorated since the age of 21 presented with complex visual hallucinations. They had begun abruptly while he was listening to music; he suddenly saw a brightly coloured circus troupe burst through the window. Thereafter he would see similar vivid animated figures on most days. Hallucinations were provoked by light and abolished by darkness or eye closure.

> A 75-year-old lady with deteriorating vision suddenly began to see brightly coloured children, animals, trees and houses. Her hallucinations occupied the entire visual field and occurred predominantly in the daytime. Though provoked by a bright light, they would persist with the eyes closed.

Dr George Paulson of Ohio State University explains:

> The major clinical features of the Charles Bonnet syndrome include a variable but usually sudden onset of complex figures. The visions are commonly those of faces, animals or flowers; or little miniature figures may be seen. The themes may be rich, the images brightly multicoloured and the impact is often described as pleasant. The most common reaction may be surprise or curiosity but rarely fear, since insight is retained with full realization of the unreality of the visions despite their striking character.

Hallucinations may also occur in up to half of those recently bereaved – and persist for up to 20 years. These 'hallucinations of widowhood' are invariably of the recently deceased, who may be heard walking up and down outside on the landing or even seen in his favourite chair, or at times be heard calling the person's name. Those who have enjoyed a happy marriage are particularly prone and indeed the opportunity to remarry is sometimes declined because of an active sense of disapproval from the late spouse. Family doctor Dewi Rees from Montgomeryshire reported one case of a 71-year-old woman who had been widowed twice and reported the confusing sensation of feeling the presence of both her late spouses in her house at the same time.

In societies that practise ancestor worship, such hallucinations are even more common. A survey of widows in Tokyo found they were virtually universal – probably because the widows actively sought to maintain links with their late husbands with daily offerings at the family altar. As one put it: 'When I want to talk to him I just light some incense. Then if I am happy I smile and show my good feelings, and if I am sad I know my tears are in his presence. When I look at a photograph of his smiling face I see he is alive, but then I look at the urn and know he is dead.'

Visual hallucinations are particlarly common amongst the Hopi Indians of North America. In a typical example described by psychiatrist Dr William Hatchett a 60-year-old woman started seeing her son (who had died from exposure) at her window. She nailed a blanket over the window – but then he took to 'visiting her every night'. She would berate him for having left her and then switch on the light, at which point her hallucination disappeared.

VISUAL ILLUSIONS

While visual hallucinations must be presumed in some way to be the brain's response to the loss of visual input from the external world, visual illusions (sometimes known as simple visual hallucinations, or photopsia) are generated from within the eye itself and take the form of striking patterns or shapes. Possible explanations are considered in the following cases:

Spider's Web

Query Mrs E.B. from Dunstable writes:

> When I wake during the night I see a *stippled spider's web pattern* across my entire field of vision. I only see this when the level of light in the bedroom is low, for example lit by a distant landing light and best against something white such as a ceiling or bedroom door. The pattern lasts for only a short time and fades as I become fully awake and move about.

Comment This spider's web pattern closely ressembles the pattern of veins across the back of the retina which, for reasons that are not at all clear, must somehow be 'projected' when the lighting is low. It may be a normal reaction, but is associated with the following condition:

♦ *Dry eye*: 'I would suggest dry eye syndrome, which can be caused by ageing or is a symptom of other medical conditions. Mrs E.B. is either looking through a dry film which breaks as she blinks or is seeing a reflection of the retina on the dry film. Having dry eyes myself and using a gel for moistening I quite often experience these – especially if the atmosphere is very dry.'

♦ *Diabetes*: 'For a number of years I have experienced a similar spider's web vision when having to go to the bathroom during the night. The pattern I 'see' should rather be described as a patchwork of changing square shapes and I believe it is something to do with the veins in the retina. I have been conscious of this pattern since I was diagnosed as being diabetic.'

♦ *Migraine*: 'I used to see very occasionally when my eyes were closed a similar spider's web pattern which lasted for perhaps a quarter for a minute. The pattern was of dark lines on a sombre background. It always took the form of a complete honeycomb lattice with two points of colour repeated, one on each side. An article in *Scientific American* included an exact illustration of the image and ascribed it to migraine and I have suffered headaches in the past.'

'The spider's web is in my opinion a form of migraine. I had a similar effect with headaches for years. Thankfully I now only get fleeting visions with no headache, usually on waking.'

Silver Ribbons

Query Mrs S.C. from Middlesex writes:

I experience a visual disturbance in my right eye whenever daylight fades and dusk sets in. It takes the form of *constant silver or white slender ribbons* or streamers on the right-hand side of my right eye, falling rapidly from the top to the bottom of the eye. If I switch on the electric light the trouble is not apparent.

Comment This may be due to 'tugging' of the vitreous humour within the eyeball on the retina.

♦ 'I have had the same silver or white ribbons or streamers. My optician said it was "retinal tug" caused by the fluid in the eye shrinking as one ages. It might continue or go spontaneously. It can lead to a detached retina.'

There are a further three visual illusions for which no satisfactory explanation was provided:

Black Shadows

Query Mrs M.J. from Aberdeen writes:

For some time I have seen *large black shadows* which come towards my eyes and then away again. They are edged with light and in the middle are changing shapes of fluorescent purple and yellow, also a small dot of fluorescent yellow darts towards my right eye as if it is going to pierce it. This all happens in the dark with my eyes open or closed. I have always suffered with migraine and the visual disturbances associated with it.

Parallel Lines

Query Mr C.G. from Cardiff writes:

I have had the following visual disturbances which can occur at any time even when I am resting and without warning. I have had a retinal detachment in the past. Quite frequently there is the appearance of several short parallel black lines, nine or ten in number, close together. There is sometimes a variation of this when I can see a single line of joined-up small loops. I can also see a line of lower case black letters, which although clearly seen as distinct letters do not form themselves into words. Most recently there has been the appearance of a circle, sometimes two circles, consisting of dense patterns of what I can best describe as tiny blue flower petals on a white background.

Shimmering Light

Query Mr K.B. from Hereford who has cataracts and a past history of glaucoma, reports the following:

Either eye can be affected, but never both at the same time. *It starts as a tiny zig-zag circle of shimmering light in the centre of my vision* and during the course of approximately twenty minutes gradually enlarges until it eventually disappears beyond the periphery of my vision. *As it grows it may alter shape slightly* and there is always a small gap in the circle which conforms closely to a capital letter C or G. The image is there whether my eyes are open or shut and is superimposed on anything I am looking at. Over the years I have told three different doctors at the Eye Hospital about this image but none of them have offered an explanation.

REVERSE TELESCOPE (MICROPSIA)

Query 64-year-old retired civil, servant Mr D.L. from Chertsey writes:

When young, about 11 years old, I was lying in bed ill, perhaps with flu or one of the many bad colds I got with living and going to school on Tyneside during and after the war. I remember *seeing one or both of my parents at the foot of the bed looking very small and distant* together with the rest of the bedroom furnishings that I could see. I don't think this lasted very long, no more than a few minutes, but I think it occurred more than once. My son was still at school and moderately ill in bed when he too mentioned seeing things looking very small.

Comment This is known as micropsia (literally 'seeing small') or the Alice in Wonderland syndrome in deference to Alice, who famously changed size. The nature of the underlying distortion is not clear, but it can be induced by defects all along the visual pathways.

- ♦ *Hereditary*: There is an hereditary form of the condition, as it runs in families. 'I used to experience it a lot when I was a child and be very frightened by it. It always happened in bed before I went to sleep and I would try and not let it happen. The strange thing was the experience was still there inside my head even when I had my eyes shut. My father said he used to experience it in French lessons in school, the teacher's head would be reduced to the size of a pin. He had been fascinated by the experience.'
- ♦ *Associated with fever*: This is probably the commonest reason, which, as with Mr D.L., only seems to occur in children.
- ♦ *Migraine*: During a migraine attack, the arteries to the back of the retina become narrow and this presumably accounts for the micropsia distortions of a migrainous attack. Lewis Carroll, author of *Alice in Wonderland*, was a migraine sufferer and Alice's dreams of being either very tall or unusually short were presumably based on his own experience. Migraine is classically associated with a headache but can – as in the following example – also induce abdominal symptoms and vomiting. 'When I was about six or seven I often used to have bilious attacks. I was usually taken into my parents' bed on these occasions and *noticed that the furniture in their room appeared to be small* and my parents looked like dolls' house inhabitants. Though I am now nearly 70 I often think of those occasions partly because I am still living in

the same house and the same furniture is still in the same room.'

♦ *Epilepsy*: The electrical disturbances in the brain of an epileptic attack can, when it involves the visual cortex, also be responsible. 'When I was between six and ten years old this occurred regularly with me. The setting was often the meal table when everything went 'a long way off' as I clearly remember calling the sensation. My parents were rather unsympathetic Victorians, I was an only child and the episodes were dismissed sharply. It also happened a few times in school, when again I dare not mention it to anyone least of all the teacher. There was a distinct feeling along with these episodes as if I was somewhat detached from myself. When eighteen months ago I was diagnosed as having epilepsy I felt the sensation of those episodes when they began was very similar to the onset of micropsia.'

♦ *Dreams*: Micropsia can also occur in dreams. 'These were bad dreams and could perhaps accurately be termed a nightmare. They took place not infrequently when I was very young and the last occasion was when I was 13 or 14. The main feature was the apparent distance of close objects (or people, who were often my parents) but they also seemed to oscillate quickly from being apparently distant to being close.

♦ *Reading*: Micropsia can also occur after prolonged reading and here the defect probably lies in the shape of the lens – for, as will be seen, it can be readily corrected.

  • 'I had a similar experience when, after late-night reading in bed, my eyes were very tired. Everything in my bedroom became far away and consequently small. In the morning all was quite normal.'

  • 'As I recall, the occurrence of this visual distortion was usually associated with excess reading, when the book would suddenly appear very small, as if at a great distance. Resting the eyes would usually cure the problem in a short time.'

- 'I have found two ways to return my vision to "normal" and thought they may help others. The first is to go for a walk and look to the middle or far distance. It also works if you look out of a window with a view, although the transition from focusing on the outside to the inside can take time. The second method is to put your hand, with fingers slightly apart over your face, and then try and focus solely on something about one centimetre away. You then gradually remove your fingers and then your head further from the object.'

MACROPSIA

There is another related visual distortion which goes to the opposite extreme, when everything seems to be very large. This, appropriately enough, is called macropsia. Not infrequently the two can alternate.

- ♦ 'I was afraid of the dark and had a night light. *I would suddenly realize the bedroom had gone very small and distant or extremely large and as though about to come down and crush me.* I would cry and my mother would come. If the main light was turned on the experience would end. It was very frightening and I dreaded it.'
- ♦ 'As a child I suffered from a similar sensation, except the effect was that if I was holding *a pencil, for example, it would feel as if it was of massive proportions* even though when looking at it, it was obvious that this was not the case.'
- ♦ 'When I was about ten I had a bad case of measles. Sometimes when I was dozing or about to go to sleep my hands and arms would appear either very small and distant or assume huge proportions. I also seem to remember that it was associated with a physical sinking feeling. It was most unpleasant and scary but could be stopped, when I no longer had measles, by a conscious effort.'
- ♦ 'As a child between the ages of six and 14 when in bed with a fever I frequently had the sensation of *being*

squashed under an enormous grey elephantine block, like clay. All the time I would be trying to get out from under it but could not.'

Hearing

Hearing, unlike vision, is much less prone to being distorted by hallucinations or illusions. The following two mysteries are, however, of considerable interest.

LOW FREQUENCY NOISE (LFN)

Query 88-year-old former hospital caterer, Mrs B.M. from Norwich, writes:

> I am one of a minority of people sensitive to low frequency noise. Gas turbines are one of my worst troubles, switching on presumably automatically when needed where the noise gradually builds up to a maximum, then after *two or three hours of the steady penetrating drone*, they switch off and very gradually run down. This regularly happens four times in the 24 hours at various hours of the day or night. I go to bed early with one sleeping tablet and I am wakened between 3.00 and 4.00 a.m. with no more sleep for two and a half to three hours.

Comment This sensitivity to low frequency noise is not unusual and indeed there is even an association for those afflicted by it. Mr Basil Tate, a recording engineer from Cornwall, makes the following observations:

> ♦ My wife has always been extraordinarily sensitive to sub-sonic sounds that the human is not supposed to hear! I am a musician and recording engineer so I like to think I know a bit about sound, but it always amazes me how my wife can *feel* ultra-low frequency sounds which are a long way away and find them extremely painful on occasions. We used to live right on the edge of the Atlantic here in Cornwall and she would sometimes lie in bed in the morning and say that she could hear a very loud

sound in her pillow. I would look out the window and see a ship on the horizon. You wouldn't believe it was possible to 'hear' at that distance but she was never wrong. There is not a lot that can be done about it, as the lower the frequency of the sound the more difficult it is to shut out. It will travel through solid walls.

Several other readers gave similar accounts:

♦ 'I live in a cottage surrounded by fields at a distance about half a mile as the crow flies from a pumping station on the local sewage system. This regularly disturbs me at night when it switches itself on and off.'

♦ 'My house is situated on the outskirts of a town and my bedroom overlooks fairly open country eight miles away. The village of Stathorpe is about five miles away, where there used to be an electricity generating station on the bank of the river Trent. Most of the year I kept the window open at night and was often bothered in the early morning by a very subdued but persistent hum, which I eventually concluded came from the turbines in the station. The more one tried to ignore it the worse it became and it could keep me awake for an hour or more. It was more noticeable on some nights than others and my observations revealed the direction of the wind made quite a difference. Then a few years later the power station was closed down, from that moment I had no further trouble.'

♦ 'Some years ago when acid house parties were the rage, there was one held about two miles from here, which raged all night and well into the next morning. While the rest of the family slept, I was demented by the deep sound of the beat and for some days after I felt quite depressed. I still find this sort of beat disturbing when I hear it coming from passing cars.'

Suggested preventive measures Most of those afflicted by sensitivity to LFN will at some time seek the help of the environmental health officer – but regrettably their powers in this situation are limited. The following suggestions have been made.

(i) *Change position of the bed*: Rooms can resonate a particular frequency and in doing so set up standing waves. These lead to points in the room where the noise is at a maximum and other places where it is at a minimum (anti-nodes and nodes). Those afflicted should move around the room at pillow height to find a position where they can put the bed (and pillow) where the noise is least. When the sound is transmitted to the house as a vibration then it is advisable to stand each leg on a thick pile of felt, say small squares about 4cms thick.

(ii) *Sony Walkman*: 'I have tried everything to cut out this noise, wax and foam earplugs, ear defenders from the Noise Abatement Society and noiseplugs from the Hearing Aid Clinic at the local hospital. I consulted a noise insulation specialist about soundproofing my bedroom and was told I could spend a lot of money but he couldn't guarantee it would cut out low frequency noise. I have now bought myself a Walkman. I tune in to the radio so as to produce a rushing noise and go to bed with earphones over my ears. I have found this to be the only solution.'

(iii) *Ventaxia fan*: 'We finally defeated the problem completely by installing a Ventaxia fan of the reversed type – i.e. drawing in filtered outside air instead of extracting. External noises are completely suppressed by the acceptable hum of the fan. It takes a little time to adjust to it, then it becomes almost hypnotic.'

EAR CLICK

Loud clicking within the ear is a most disabling complaint. Besides the tormenting noise, those afflicted usually have difficulty concentrating and sleeping. The mechanism involves a spasm of the muscle that controls the soft palate at the back of the throat, which in turn causes the narrow eustachian tube to the middle ear to snap open and shut. Dr Gunther Deuschel, neurologist at the University of Freiburg in Germany, describes a typical case: 'A 53-year-old man complained of a *right-sided ear click* that seriously interfered with his work as a civil servant. His sleep was severely disturbed. Physical examination was normal except for tremor of the soft palate and synchronous ear clicks that could be heard at a distance of about one metre.'

Treatment The favoured treatment is botulinum toxin, that paralyses the nerve responsible for the tremor of the palate. This usually leads to cessation of the click within a couple of days, though the toxin can cause – as a side-effect – mild nasal regurgitation of fluids when drinking rapidly. This can be readily controlled and is more than offset by the ability to have a full night's sleep again.

Sometimes ear clicking can be associated with wiggling ears, as described in the following case:

A 69-year-old woman had a long history of frequent wiggling of her left ear – often aggravated by emotional distress. She could neither voluntarily suppress these movements nor could she ever deliberately wiggle her ears. She had also had a more recent history of a regular clicking sound more pronounced in the left than in the right ear. An injection of the relevant muscle with botulinum toxin alleviated the ear movement.

There are two further mysteries for which no satisfactory explanations were offered.

INTERMITTENT DEAFNESS

Query Mrs H.E. from Wimbledon writes:

My husband *experiences the onset of deafness in one ear usually with an accompanying ringing sound (similar to tinnitus) every time we visit an art gallery or museum.* Most recently it happened as we were approaching the gallery to see an exhibition of the works of Goya. Weird or what? It happens in both modern buildings and old ones. It drives him mad. We call it 'gallery ear'. At home, or anywhere else – theatres, railway stations, etc – he is OK.

THROBBING EAR

Query Mr B.J. from Richmond writes:

> When I am using the telephone, if I hold the receiver to my right ear, *the voice of the other party provokes an unpleasant intermittent throbbing, like bubbles bursting in my left ear.* I transfer the receiver to my left ear, the throbbing stops. In the recent past the same throbbing, also in my left ear, would start in bed if I lay on my left side with my ear on the pillow. It was extremely disturbing and would force me to turn on to my right side. However, this particular manifestation has not recurred for several months.

Another reader comments: 'I too for many years have noticed a slight "thudding" noise corresponding exactly to speech when on the telephone or listening to the radio via an earpiece. It is, however, only my left ear which is affected – the right is fine.'

Taste and Smell

The sensations of taste and smell are very closely related, as taste is primarily perceived through the sense of smell in the nose. Imagine, for example, you are enjoying a plate of steak and chips and a glass of claret. The odour molecules from the claret percolate up through the nose where they come across millions of minute hairs on the surface of the olfactory or smelling nerve. These hairs are studded with receptors into which the odour molecules fit like a lock and a key, thus initiating nerve impulses to the taste sensors in the brain. Simultaneously, the odour molecules released by chewing on the steak and chips are passed up through the back of the mouth into the nose, where they come across their own appropriate receptors, so the impression of the taste of steak is also mediated by the same route. This major contribution of the sense of smell to taste becomes obvious during a heavy cold which causes both a loss of smell and an inability to taste food and drink.

By comparison, the contribution of the taste buds in the mouth to taste is quite limited, with only four main types being recognized – salt, sour, sweet and bitter – evenly distributed around the tongue and palate. Their primary purpose is less to do with the appreciation of food than to serve more basic physiological functions – thus the 'salt' taste buds are highly sensitive to the amount of salt in the body and induce a craving for the mineral if the blood becomes salt depleted.

The problems that may affect the sensations of taste and smell are therefore not surprisingly quite similar, both being due to an abnormality of the functioning of the nerves, which may follow a viral infection or come out of the blue for no apparent reason. This results in the loss of the sense of smell or taste (or both) or alternatively – and worse – a foul sensation in the mouth, or an exaggeration of one or other of the primary taste types so everything tastes too salty, too sweet or too metallic.

LOSS OF SMELL (ANOSMIA)

Loss of smell or anosmia may be due to damage to the olfactory (smelling) nerve following a bad cold or a bout of sinusitis, or following a head injury. A doctor describes the condition as it affected his wife:

My wife is anosmic. It happened after an acute respiratory tract infection. She came out of it cheerful and fit except for having lost her sense of smell. At first she regarded this as merely a nuisance and was comforted by our doctor's assurance that with the passage of time (unspecified) all the odours of this world would be hers to enjoy once again. Weeks went by in which she sniffed experimentally at this and that but without results.

One day she came in very excited. While passing a farm she had actually identified the unmistakable aroma of pig manure. Shortly after *she began to find that a few ordinary objects had an odour, but always the same odour: 'old wet biscuits'*. The intensity of the beastly biscuit smell is slowly increasing and my wife does not care for it at all. She has reached a stage of resignation, but I remain upset and interrupted. She calls me to the kitchen to sniff at sauces or stuffing. She ignores the exotically scented paper white narcissi I have cultivated. She no longer dabs on the costly perfume I gave her, quite disregarding that it had been bought mainly for my pleasure.

Treatment With luck the sense of smell will eventually return, but in the meantime there is not much that can be done. The following two options have been suggested, however:

(i) *Steroids*: Dr Alan Knight of Toronto, who developed anosmia following an acute attack of sinusitis, describes the benefits of steroids: 'Anosmia can be treated by reducing the inflammation. This is easily and safely done by a short course of oral steroids such as prednisolone. Adverse effects are uncommon. These should be followed by long-term topical steroid nasal sprays. Sadly the sense may gradually decline and require a repeat treatment. I save it for the Christmas turkey and a good claret.'

(ii) *Theophyllines*: Dr Robert Hankin of the Taste and Smell Clinic in Washington writes: 'Theophylline 250–750mg daily in divided doses has, in selected patients with anosmia, permanently restored smell function to or towards normal. Six to 18 weeks of therapy may be necessary.'

SWEET SMELL

Sometimes rather than a complete loss of smell, one particular form becomes dominant, as descibed here:

♦ 'Since my husband's death from a stroke I have had a *sickly scented smell* in my nostrils. I awaken during the night with it and my urine, which is perfectly normal, has the same scented smell. I do not have diabetes. My smell is perfectly normal in other respects except when chopping onions I no longer smell them, whereas before I used to have tears rolling down my face.'

♦ 'I am currently suffering from a *hypersensitivity to a fusty-sweet smell/flavour* emanating from certain foods which most people seem unaware of, at least until it reaches high concentration. It causes nausea and lack of appetite. I first encountered it in the summer on imported celery, fennel, peaches and nectarines. It has spread considerably to other foodstuffs since then.'

METALLIC TASTE

An unpleasant metallic taste – like old pennies – may occur alone or as part of a more generalized mouth disorder.

Query 80-year-old Mrs A.D. from Wiltshire writes: 'For the last year I have had the *most unpleasant metallic taste* in my mouth with a constant sense of dryness, as if my salivary glands are no longer working.'

Comment Most frequently dry mouth is another sign of ageing – in this case the drying up of the glands that produce the saliva that keeps the mouth moist. It may be a side-effect of certain drugs, particularly those used in the treatment of depression and raised blood pressure. Alternatively it can be part of a more generalized drying up of the mucous membranes known as the sicca (dry) syndrome most commonly associated with Sjogren's syndrome, so named after the Swedish ophthalmologist who first described it. The fungal infection thrush can also cause dry mouth.

Treatment

(i) Dry mouth and metallic taste

♦ *Campari*: 'Several years ago after a severe stomach upset I suffered from dry mouth. It is extremely difficult to eat anything as you need a cup of water or Guinness with each mouthful. I lost weight amazingly and looked as if I had just come out of Belsen. Eventually one of my sons came to stay and produced a solution to the problem – he had been chatting about it with another sufferer, a man who had travelled in Italy and had been given a cure by an Italian barman. It is a shot of Campari, softened in its bitterness by the addition of two or three times as much lime juice cordial or other fruit flavour, topping up to a tumblerful with plain water. Drink once a day. I tried it out of desperation and was amazed at its success. I have never again had the problem of a dry mouth and gradually got back my normal weight.'

♦ *Linen thread*: 'I contracted Sjogren's syndrome and for many years it almost drove me crazy, until I adopted the following tip for the alleviation of my dry mouth. I obtained considerable relief by placing in my mouth a length of linen thread about three inches long (cotton thread will do, not manmade fibres). I think the thread (which I knot at both ends to prevent it from unwinding) absorbs such saliva as does come down through the salivary glands until it becomes quite soggy thus providing good lubrication in the mouth.'

♦ *Antifungal drugs*: 'I experienced a dry mouth and a metallic taste a while back and kept hoping it would go away. Some days it would be a bit better than others. I was prescribed vitamin pills, throat sprays, lozenges. Nothing worked. Eventually a throat consultant diagnosed 'a very severe fungal infection'. He gave me five tablets of Diflucan to combat the problem, instructing me to see my family doctor if the infection returned. It did, some months later, but this time only one tablet was prescribed and that worked.'

(ii) Metallic taste alone

When the metallic taste occurs alone the following possibilities may be considered:

♦ *Drug side-effects*: Many drugs can cause metallic taste as a side-effect, including the antibiotics Metronidazole and Tetracycline and local anaesthetics such as Lignocane.

♦ *Food sensitivity*: 'I describe my taste as iron, which I experience on the rare occasions when I eat cheese. I normally eat Flora margarine, but when we decided to have a change I got the same taste from butter – not immediately but by the end of a half pound pack and also after eating cream. I cannot drink Ribena Light or any lemonades containing artificial sweeteners. The culprit, it transpired, was a lipstick to which I was allergic. I am now extremely careful which lipstick I use, as I have had the odd lapse which has responded to changing the lipstick.'

♦ *Metallic fillings*: Metal fillings develop a natural protective coating, which can be removed by over-enthusiastic brushing, exposing new, bare metal which you can then taste. Sometimes two different metals e.g. gold and silver, react to each other setting up a small electric circuit that dissolves the metal in the mouth. 'I had a very nasty metallic taste in my mouth until my fillings were carefully replaced with non-metallic composite. I know this is a very controversial area amongst dentists, but know of a large number of people whose health dramatically improved once amalgams had been removed.'

♦ *Serious underlying medical problems*: Very occasionally a metallic taste in the mouth can be the first sign of some serious underlying medical condition:

• 'I am concerned that a dry mouth with a metallic taste may indicate some form of malignancy of the gastro-intestinal tract.'

• 'Without wishing to be pessimistic I had a metallic taste in my mouth for about six months before a diagnosis of ovarian cancer was made.'

• 'I had a very nasty metallic taste with nausea and was eventually diagnosed as having kidney failure.'

There is no specific treatment to counteract the metallic taste, though one reader recommends 'powdered ginger on meals and bananas'. Alternatively, 'Chewing gum is my life saver, though I hate using it when in public. It seems to disguise the awful background taste, though with lengthy use I end up suffering from jaw ache!'

SWEET/SALTY TASTE

Query 54-year-old Mrs S.C. from Kent writes: 'I have a *horrid salty taste* in my mouth about which I have consulted my family doctor three or four times to no avail. It seems to get worse at different times of the month and the edges of my tongue can feel quite sore although there is nothing to see. I assure you it is most unpleasant.'

Query Mrs M.L. from Carmarthenshire writes: 'I have a curious complaint. My trouble is *a very sweet taste* in my mouth. It is all right in the morning, but builds up during the day until it is almost unbearable by the evening. It does not seem to make any difference if I eat sweet things or not. I was tested for diabetes some years ago, but the result was negative.'

Comment These abnormalities of sensation have been compared to the phantom pains following leg amputation where the sensory nerves generate garbled or distorted messages. Dr Robert Hankin of the Taste and Smell Clinic in Washington observes:

> Those affected find themselves at the mercy of the abormal taste, which can become the dominant controlling factor in their lives, limiting their sociability. Some feel that eating or chewing with repeated use of snacks, candies, gum or mints modifies the abormal taste, but this can cause weight gain or teeth problems. Some brush their teeth or use mouthwashes multiple times a day which may temporarily alleviate the symptoms, but it always returns.

Treatment With luck the taste abnormality will improve spontaneously but the following possibilities should be considered.

(i) *Overwhelming the abnormal sensation*: 'The answer is about three teaspoonfuls of salt, partially dissolved in a cup of quite hot water and swilled round the mouth so as to reach every nook and cranny. Hold it in the mouth until the salt solution cools down, then spit out. Repeat until cup is empty. This has to be done two or three times a day and at bedtime. It tastes pretty unpleasant and makes your mouth feel dry and salty but it is not as bad as the original complaint.'

(ii) *Drug medication*: Dr Hankin writes: 'The symptoms can be considered a variant of oral pain, where excess activity of the receptors for the neurotransmitter dopamine have been implicated. Accordingly counteracting drugs such as Haloperidol, Thioridazine or Pimozide have been useful.

FOUL TASTE (DYSGEUSIA)

A persistent foul taste in the mouth is a debilitating disorder which may be associated with poor dental hygiene, sinusitis, the use of antidepressant medication, stroke and kidney failure. Most commonly, however, it is a solitary symptom affecting the nerves of taste. Dr Robert Hankin describes a case:

A 53-year-old white male pizza maker experienced the sudden onset of severe upper respiratory tract infection. At the time he noted the sudden loss of ability to taste and smell which persisted after recovery from the acute illness. On the journey to work at the restaurant *he noted a profound almost overpoweringly obnoxious odour associated with various foods and vapours.* Any attempt to eat these foods was associated with an *overpoweringly obnoxious taste.* He described the odour of foods as rotten, as if they smelt and taste like manure or decaying garbage. The foods which produced these symptoms included meat, eggs, fish, cheeses, bread, coffee, tomatoes and other spices. He also complained of a persistent sour, bitter, metallic taste in his mouth which never diminished in intensity and a 'rotten' smell was similarly persistent in his nose.

Dr Christine Lawrence of the Albert Einstein College of Medicine in New York experienced this foul taste as a complication of an infection that had involved the nerves to the tongue.

One morning I *awoke with a foul taste* and assumed that the crowned molar was the source. My dentist assured me that all my teeth were in good condition. The foul taste persisted and eventually I returned insisting that something was 'rotting' in my mouth and I requested he remove the crown. He was confident the crown was not the source and urged me to delay, which I did.

The taste was often so bad I was unable to eat and avoided standing close to others so as to spare them the [imaginary] offensive odour. The perverted taste ranged from awful to repulsive. After three years, the vile sensation finally waned, although it recurred briefly several times, but lack of discrimination of taste has persisted. Foregoing the pleasure of lingering over a tasty meal was sad in itself, but after years of dysgeusia, it seemed a minor loss.

Treatment Two-thirds of patients will improve spontaneously within a couple of years. There is no effective remedy, though there are reports that if it occurs around the menopause oestrogen is helpful, as are zinc supplements – even in the presence of normal zinc levels.

4
Headache

There are numerous causes of headache, most of which are a feature of some common ailment such as flu or sinusitis which are easy enough to ascertain, or can be diagnosed by appropriate investigations such as blood tests or X-rays. We consider here interesting or unusual presentations of one or other of the primary types of headache – migraine, tension, cluster or continuous headaches and a miscellany of others.

'HANGOVER' MIGRAINE

Query Physicist, Dr J.J. from Bucks writes:

> I am a very modest drinker but periodically have a *hangover-like feeling* which comes and goes without apparent reason. The *feeling is usually centred on the nasal area and is often associated with a slight sore throat in the hard palate area.* At its worst it is difficult to do anything other than rest with the eyes shut. At other times I can force myself to ignore it. Typically I have three or four attacks for about a week or two each per year, but sometimes much longer. The attacks themselves may last from a few minutes to hours. I also have periods of remission lasting up to six months.

Comment Dr Pauley from Colchester writes:

> My suspicion is that this man is suffering from migraine. The long remissions, 'hangover' feelings and duration of attacks all fit.

The classic migrainous headache occupies one side of the head and is associated with vomiting and an aversion to light. It may be associated with an 'aura' of visual hallucinations or sensations of pins and needles in the limbs. But migraine is also a frequent cause of 'mystery' syndromes. Attacks involve first a constriction then dilation of blood vessels so when the blood supply to the balance centre in the brain is involved, this results in dizziness. If the vessels to the gut are involved this results in abdominal pain and nausea and so on. Here it would seem the symptoms are due to blood vessels of the nasal area accounting for the 'hangover-like' feeling. The difficulty in making the diagnosis and identifying the underlying cause – such as case food sensitivity – is illustrated by the following:

> I have had 'hangovers' for more than 20 years, despite giving up alcohol altogether, and have seen all manner of medical specialists and alternative therapists. I eventually, against my better judgement, attended a nutritional clinic where I was found to be sensitive to wheat, barley and oats. These I duly excluded from my diet and my recovery has been nothing short of a miracle.

BUZZING, FLUTTERING, DAILY (TENSION) HEADACHE

Mrs D.K. from Wales writes on behalf of her 53-year-old husband:

> For the last 18 months my husband has had *daily headaches that come on late in the day* – but never prevent him sleeping at night. He describes them as a *buzzing, fluttering sensation that grows into a constant pain.* We can identify no link with food or lifestyle that dictates this pattern. It does not disappear on holiday. A brain scan revealed no abnormality and eventually a neurologist diagnosed the condition as 'cramp of the scalp muscles'. An alcoholic drink provides half an hour's respite – as does a hot shower on his scalp or massage. Alternatively, wearing a tight sweat band round his forehead and then removing it appears to be his best option.

Comment Tension headaches are the commonest of all types where the sensation of pressure pulling on the top of the head is attributed to spasm of the scalp muscles. It may be precipitated by stressful situations, but the precise underlying cause remains obscure. Neurologist Dr John Patten comments:

> A typical acute tension headache starts as a tight feeling at the back of the scalp and then spreads over the head as a 'tight' feeling. Similar headaches occur towards the end of each day. When the headaches continue to occur on a daily basis they are classified as 'chronic tension headaches'. The most effective treatment is Amitriptyline in a dose of 10–50mg at night.'

HOT POKER (CLUSTER) HEADACHE

Query Mrs F.M. from Salcombe writes:

> For the past six years I have been suffering with headaches that nearly always follow the same pattern – I wake in the morning with a *slight throbbing pain over my left eye; gradually this increases and eventually* (after a few hours) *the pain has included the whole of the left side of the back of my head and throat*. It is worse if I bend or lie down, if I am in an enclosed atmosphere or if I drink alcohol. After about 36 hours the pain subsides and eventually disappears. These headaches occur every 10–14 days and are always accompanied by a *blocked up nose*. I have tried everything I can think of, but can get no relief. Four years ago I consulted a specialist who suggested an operation for a deviated septum of the nose might do the trick. I had the operation but it made not the slightest difference.

Comment Mr W.G. Collington, ophthalmologist from Newcastle writes:

> I have no doubt this lady is suffering from cluster headaches, otherwise known as periodic migrainous neuralgia. Cluster headaches are so called because they tend to be grouped in a series for weeks or months, interrupted by equally prolonged symptom-free intervals. Often the clusters return at the same time each year. The severe pain is often described as '*a hot poker' penetrating one eye* and is experienced from once every other day to eight times daily. The side of the head on which the pain is felt can vary between attacks but it almost never occurs on both sides at the same time. In contrast to migraine, where the sufferer only wishes to lie still

and quiet in a dark room, the patient with a cluster migraine cannot stay still but must pace uncontrollably up and down. Although the diagnosis should not be difficult, there may be associated symptoms such as eye redness and nasal congestion or a runny nose, which may suggest the problem lies in the sinuses or elsewhere.

Many years may pass before the correct diagnosis is made, as the following account from a reader described:

My own cluster headaches were extensively investigated for more than 20 years and diagnosed as neuritis, sinusitis, trigeminal neuralgia interspersed with many consultations with ENT and dental departments. The big breakthrough came when I was having dinner with friends, my host was a professor of surgery and the other guest was a consultant physician. After a mouthful of red wine I began a full-blown attack. The physican gave a ball-by-ball commentary, accurately forecasting the next stage. It was a very edifying episode and for the first time it gave me an accurate diagnosis.

Treatment Precipitants should be avoided – as in the case outlined above, red wine – but others include the food additive MSG, often added to fast foods, and sulphur dioxide. This can be found in white wine, meringue pie, muesli and frozen fish pie. Some sufferers report that changes in altitude and air travel, as well as strong sunlight and changes in sleep pattern, are potential triggers of cluster attacks.

Painkillers usually do not work rapidly enough to stop the pain once it has started. The anti-migraine drug Ergotamine can be helpful. The local anaesthetic Lidocaine, administered as nose drops directly into the nostril on the affected side, can abort an attack. Finally, for reasons that are not clear, breathing pure oxygen from a tank at the onset of an attack can lead to relief within 15 minutes:

I got the necessary oxygen equipment and when the next cluster occurred I found an attack could be totally abated within three to five minutes. With more experience I discovered that my using oxygen as soon as an attack was signalled (usually by a bout of yawning) I could abort an attack. Clusters have become less frequent and less severe.

CONTINUOUS HEMICRANIAL ('HALF HEAD') HEADACHE

In Chapter 1, Dr Nick Fox, specialist registrar in neurology in London, illustrated both the difficulties that can be encountered in determining the cause of headache and the absolute importance of doing so in permitting appropriate treatment to be instituted. His patient was a 50-year-old deaf mute woman who had suffered from headache for 40 years which had been misdiagnosed as migraine:

> Slowing and laboriously she 'drew' her headache for me – it was *continuous but fluctuated between 9/10 and 10/10 where 10/10 was the worst pain she had ever had. It was always left sided and never across the mid line.* None of the migraine treatments had helped. The history now sounded like hemicrania continua in which case the headache should respond to Indomethacin. She agreed to try it.
>
> Four weeks later she looked transformed. She handed me a note explaining her pain was better than it had been for 40 years – again she had 'drawn' the pain. It now scored 1/10.

Dr Lawrence Newman of the Albert Einstein College of Medicine in New York comments: 'It is difficult to explain the unique benefits of Indomethacin and the relative lack of benefits of other drugs. Response is rapid, usually developing in a matter of hours. Many patients report that delaying or skipping a single dose of the medication can result in prompt recurrence of the headache.'

HYPNIC (SLEEPING) HEADACHE

This, as the name suggests, afflicts the sufferer at night often several times and responds to the drug Lithium, as Dr Newman again reports:

> An 84-year-old woman had a two-year history of *diffuse pulsating headaches* which wakened her from sleep every night, usually three times. Each headache lasted approximately 30 minutes and recurred at two-hour intervals. She was never wakened by headache during her daily afternoon nap. She had been treated with

numerous medications to no avail. All investigations including CT scan had been normal. She was treated with lithium carbonate 300mg at bedtime, and over a period of two weeks the headaches occurred later each night or upon waking in the morning. The dose was then increased to 600mg and she had a sustained remission for two months. When treatment was discontinued she had a prompt recurrence of her headaches.

FLEETING HEADACHE (CEPHALGIA FUGAX)

This is described as a *sharp, stabbing, darting or shooting pain that usually lasts for a split second* and rarely for more than a minute. Its frequency ranges from five times a day to once a week. It is also known, for obvious reasons, as the 'icepick headache'.

Dr Edward Martin, consultant neurologist at St Vincent's Hospital, Dublin, in his survey of 37 patients, reports that in ten the headache improved spontaneously within a year. In the remainder the symptoms persisted intermittently and there is no known treatment.

COITAL HEADACHE

This headache occurs during sexual intercourse, though its sudden onset and explosive nature suggests to the sufferer that some catastophic event has occurred such as haemorrhage into the brain. A similar ferocious headache can be induced by any form of exertion. Dr Mark Porter of the Texas Medical Centre describes a typical case:

A 40-year-old man had a two-year history of *intermittent coital headaches occurring abruptly at orgasm* or just seconds before. The headache was *severe with throbbing pain at the back of the skull lasting 5–30 minutes.* They occurred with marital and during extra-marital sexual intercourse. Fatigue, stress, kneeling position and particularly intense orgasms made the headaches worse. Propranolol 120mg a day resulted in complete relief. After three weeks he discontinued the medication and the headaches promptly returned.

COUGH HEADACHE

The development of a *pounding headache at the back of the skull after coughing* may indicate that the brain stem is slipping through the hole at the base of the skull, which may require surgery. British neurologist Dr Bernard Williams describes the case of a 27-year-old 'slender and intelligent woman':

> She would have a pounding headache if she suddenly stood up after lying or sitting. It seldom lasted more than a minute. Laughing, coughing and straining were painful. She managed by moving slowly when getting up. She would, when getting out of bed, roll to the edge of the bed, lower her legs to the floor until she was kneeling then gradually stand. The pain could sometimes be relieved by stooping forwards and flexing the head.
>
> Investigations revealed protrusion of the brain stem through the opening or foramen magnum at the base of the skull and the anatomical defect was closed at operation. Subsequent to the operation there has been no recurrence of the headache and she gave birth normally to a child a year later.

TURTLE HEADACHE

Turtle headaches occur in those who on waking desire to return back to sleep and, finding the daylight a nuisance, pull the bedcovers over the head. When they awake for a second time, they have a *generalized headache that has been attributed to oxygen deprivation* while under the cover and an *associated compensatory accummulation of carbon dioxide in the blood*. Dr Gordon Gilbert of Florida comments: 'When the background of a turtle headache is explained to the patient, he is always quite willing to discontinue the habit responsible and the headaches immediately disappear.'

EXPLODING HEAD

Query 74-year-old Mrs E.D. from Warrington writes: 'Often when on my left side in the sleep position *my head has an* *explosion*. It occurs as far as I can tell above my left ear often in close succession for one or two nights and then goes away.'

Comment This phenomenon is known – for obvious reasons – as exploding head syndrome. It has also been described in the following ways:

♦ 'As if my head was bursting with a flash of lightning after which I will be dazed for a split second and will come round terrified, my heart thumping. There is no pain, just a frightening sense of explosion.'
♦ 'It is more of a thunderclap than a pain, though you would never know when it is coming except that it is always when you are asleep.'
♦ 'I liken the spasms to mini explosions and small bursts of air or violent electric buzzes. They did happen on wakening but more often woke me suddenly in the night. They left me feeling washed out.'

Consultant neurologist Dr J.M.S. Pearce observes:

Patients are so alarmed at first they may inaccurately describe it as a pain but closer questioning shows the awareness is not of a hurt, but of a noise in the centre or back of the head. The syndrome is entirely benign and I suspect common. The cause of the problem remains a mystery. Firm reassurance is essential but drug therapy seems unwarranted.

One reader, however, relates the explosions to instability of the vertebrae in the neck: 'I believe that at some stage I changed from two pillows to having just a very thin pillow after which I developed noises in my head, dull thuds, gunshots, gongs and chimes. I was scared they were precursors to a stroke. Suddenly my head "asked" for a fatter pillow. Since using one the bangs have stopped.'

Two possible variants of exploding head syndrome have also been described.

♦ 'I am very worried about bumps inside my head. Perhaps "jerks" better describes them. As I wake in the morning I get the sensation of a sudden movement, sometimes vigorous but more often gentle. It left me feeling vaguely unwell and sometimes with a headache over my eyes.'

♦ 'I am often woken suddenly by a loud and very real noise. It may be the sound of an explosion or alternatively I have rushed to the window and looked through the curtains after hearing a tile from the roof breaking on the ground; or I have rushed out of the bedroom to answer the ringing of the phone; or the front doorbell rings and before I get used to the idea it is all in the head I would rush to open the door thinking it was a parcel delivery.'

BENIGN CEREBELLAR HYPERTENSION

A rare, but important, cause of headache is described below in the case of a teenage girl:

For some years my daughter in her late teens suffered from sessions of *excruciating head pains lasting for two or three days at a time*. They were sufficient to make her *scream out with pain, to be repeatedly sick and make sleep impossible*. They occurred roughly every three weeks. She described it *as feeling as though a steel band was being slowly tightened across her head until it was unbearable and inescapable*.

It was inevitably diagnosed as migraine and all the usual treatments prescribed along with a variety of exclusion diets. All investigations were normal. She completely collapsed in the street on several occasions becoming totally unconscious.

You can imagine we were at our wits' ends, some 20 different doctors had seen her over three years and not one arrived at a satisfactory diagnosis. At last while in hospital for yet more tests, she noticed that after a spinal tap her symptoms largely disappeared. This then led to the diagnosis of benign cerebellar hypertension – though benign is perhaps not a word that the sufferer would use to describe it. Initially a permanent shunt was proposed to drain the excess spinal fluid into the chest cavity but we were fortunate to catch a consultant virtually on his last working day before retirement who suggested cortisone. The response was miraculous and after a month of steadily reducing doses she could control the attacks with half a tablet a day. Since then we have learnt the condition affects mainly young women in their late teens and they grow out of it, which she did. She has had no further attacks after several years.

5

Facial Pain

The face is the focus of more diverse forms of sensation than any other part of the body – taste, smell, touch, sight, hearing. It thus has a particularly rich nerve supply and so is prone to an extraordinarily diverse range of 'pain syndromes'. Several have been alluded to in other sections of the book, including cluster headache, migraine headache, phantom tooth pain, Burning Mouth Syndrome and eye and ear pain. There are, of course, numerous possible causes of facial pain arising from disease or problems with the many structures of the face such as the teeth (dental caries), sinuses (sinusitis), tongue, nose and pharynx. Clearly, then, patients with facial pain have to be carefully evaluated and investigated. The assumption in what follows is that these have been done, no underlying cause has been identified and the source of the pain must be presumed to lie in the nerves themselves, the muscles or joints.

STABBING FACIAL PAIN (TRIGEMINAL NEURALGIA)

Query 1 Mrs S.G. from Yorkshire writes:

My symptoms start with *tenderness around the eye or elsewhere in the head*. In that area I then get the most *terrible jabbing pains at very frequent intervals*. I feel like a 'zombie' and am caught anticipating the next jab. I try not to move my jaw or head as this may bring on a jab in the sensitive area. This can last for up to a week, gradually fading away.

Query 2 Mrs C.S., retired nurse from West Sussex, writes:

For quite a number of years I have noticed a *'tender' sensation at the lightest tough on my left eyelid and a 'sore' feeling on turning the eye*. This 'tenderness' progresses to the left side of the face. The gums of the upper jaw molars also feel tender. The symptoms disappear after about three days. I also suffer from sharp stabbing pains of the left ear at the side of the face which are not necessarily related to the tenderness described.

Query 3 Mrs M.S. from Kent writes:

I have *intense pain on one side of my face from time to time*. Mine has no definitive starting point, but from forehead to chin and across from cheek to cheek *I can't bear the slightest touch of fingertips* and to sleep is almost impossible. I have the impression the area is hot although it isn't in fact and that there must be something visible akin to severe sunburn or scalding by steam, but the face looks normal. It generally lasts several days then fades gradually. I wonder if it is connected to the 'dormant' herpes virus which causes cold sores, of which I may get one or two a year – although there doesn't appear to be any pattern.

Comment This is trigeminal neuralgia, so called because the nerve involved has three (trigeminal) separate branches that supply the face. It was first described by the ancient Greek physician Arateaus of Cappadocia as a pain where 'spasm and distortion of the face takes place'. The philosopher and physician John Locke gives a particularly good description from 1677 in one of his patients, the Countess of Northumberland:

An attack of such violent and exquisite torment that it forced her to . . . cries and shrieks. When the attack came, there was as if a flash of fire all of a sudden shot into all those parts. Speaking was apt to put her into these attacks, sometimes opening her mouth to take anything or touching her gum.

The trigeminal, or fifth, nerve is one of 12 cranial nerves that arise from the base of the brain and supply the cranium or skull and their associated parts. Two other cranial nerves (see below) are associated with similar acute pain affecting the relevant site of the head they supply. The underlying cause is unknown, though – as we will see – in some the nerve may be being compressed by a blood vessel within the ear. Further, some patients – as Mrs M.S. from Kent – relate their episodes to an outbreak of the herpes cold virus on the face which lies dormant in the nerve periodically flaring up on the surface.

The characteristic type of pain is as described by Mrs S.B. from York, a *'sharp, terrifying lancinating pain'*, but can also take the form of a more generalized soreness. Neurologist Dr Robert Frank writes: 'The pain is typically described as shooting, sharp, burning like electricity or knife-like'. It can be precipitated by washing one's face, talking and eating (particularly pungent fruit) and brushing the hair. Cold winds and draughts, emotional stress and extremes of emotion can also precipitate attacks. Some of these can be avoided, as a reader comments:

♦ *Cold winds*: In winter and on windy days – even in the height of summer – keep your ears covered and on very cold days, cheeks too. Just one blast of cold air can be enough to trigger an attack. It is easier for women – we can wear a hat, or better still a cotton scarf, which can be pulled over the offending cheek to lessen the cold air. Men need a balaclava or hat with Sherlock Holmes-type ear flaps. Even a cotton wool earplug will help. Keep your head warm and always avoid draughts.

Treatment

(i) *Tegretol*: The principal treatment is the drug Tegretol, or carbamazepine, originally developed for the treatment of epilepsy. It probably works in a similar way by 'damping down' the electrical discharges of the nerves that are responsible for the pain.

For over three years I suffered badly with stabbing pains in my face. My dentist removed teeth in the offending area and eventually I visited the dental department of the local hospital. In desperation after many months of pain I mentioned it to my family doctor and after some thought he said, 'I've got the little fellows for you.' He prescribed Tegretol taken at bedtime. The relief was unbelievable. Needless to say I would never be without them.

(ii) *Pain-blocking injections*: For those not helped by Tegretol, there is the possibility of knocking out the nerve responsible with an appropriate injection.

I have suffered from this condition for 20 years. Early treatment with a low dose of Tegretol was not effective. I tried a course of acupuncture which only worked for a short period. I was then referred to a pain relief unit at the local hospital. The neurologist's specialty was trigeminal neuralgia and migraine. My treatment was a massive pain-blocking injection into the nerve at the base of the lower gum by the tongue which was effective for several months. Eventually because of scar tissue no further injections could be given.

(iii) *Operation*: An alternative approach is an operation to 'decompress' the nerve – that is, separate it from a blood vessel that is pressing on it which, in some cases, accounts for the syndrome.

I suffered from this miserable complaint for eight years till eventually I was put on Tegretol. It helped in some small way but with various bad side-effects. In the end I was referred to a consultant neurosurgeon at Walton Hospital, Liverpool, who performed the operation of 'microvascular decompression' and since then I have been pain free and on no medication. I can thoroughly recommend this course of action and only wish I had known of it sooner.

(iv) *The alternatives*: Several readers suggest alternative approaches to treatment.

♦ *Acupressure*: 'My son was desperately in need of help. Acupressure was brilliant. Press inwards at the inner end of the eyebrow or press downwards towards the jaw and the point near the corners of the mouth. Press lightly for 5–10 minutes and repeat hourly.'
   'Some seven years ago my trigeminal neuralgia returned. Having by that time become interested in

Chinese medicine, I pressed the pressure point on the inner eyebrow and found instant relief. I maintained a gentle pressure for five or ten minutes and the pain went and did not recur.'

♦ *Hypnosis*: 'My mother suffered from this for many years. Eventually when she was 70, during a particularly bad spell I persuaded her, against her will, to visit a hypnotist. She was very sceptical that this could help when all the experts could not and she was adamant she had not gone into a trance, so it could not possibly work. I sat in the room as the hypnotist told her that her own finger could cure her and that she could touch her face with it and watched in amazement as her finger hesitated as though it knew the pain would be intense, but then it began quite easily to stroke her nose and her cheek. After that visit she had immediate relief. We returned once more and then were given a tape by the hynotist for her to listen to if the pain returned. She never suffered again from this and died ten years later.'

♦ *Chocolate sensitivity*: 'My wife suffered from this complaint for many years and reached the point where it was clearly a case of "living with it". We began to realize that attacks seemed to occur after Christmas and the New Year, Easter and after her birthday. It seemed to me there was likely to be a connection and as these are all times of indulgence it was not unreasonable to suspect food or drink. The one thing it could be, of course, was chocolate, particularly of the plain variety and it was decided to cut it out altogether. Quite simply that has proved the complete solution. When my wife does eat a limited amount of chocolate she knows it will trigger off the neuralgia. The effect appears to build up, with quite a delay between eating it and the first twinges being felt, the severity of the attack depending on how much has been eaten. There is not the slightest doubt in her mind that this has been the cause of her neuralgia.'

♦ *Cranial osteopathy*: Practitioners qualified in cranial manipulation can offer patients relief for their symptoms by, it is claimed, releasing restrictions of the cranial sutures that may be putting mechanical strain on the trigeminal nerve.

♦ *Homeopathy*: 'I used to suffer from this dreadful imposition for years until I became interested in homeopathy. I found it could be treated with spigelia – that was simply wonderful. After two days of tablets, the pain went completely. I had another slight attack some time later which went within 24 hours of taking the tablets again. The relief is wonderful. You have no idea of the absolute agony trying to swallow anything liquid or solid. I try to keep out of draughts, however small, as these always seem to bring on an attack.

(v) *Dental treatment*: The pain of trigeminal neuralgia can be mimicked by several other conditions, most notably pain of dental origin which similarly can be lancinating, brought on by chewing and lasting for short periods. There is usually, however, a background discomfort and the symptoms are not clearly demarcated into one or other divisions of the nerves.

♦ 'I suffered from similar symptoms for many years until my dentist sent me to a specialist to X-ray the area affected and discovered an impacted wisdom tooth which was growing sideways into another tooth. I had the impacted tooth removed and since then I have been pain free.'

♦ 'I have had one patient with very similar symptoms, so much so he was scheduled for an injection of the facial nerve on the affected side. He did, however, have an upper molar on that side which had been root treated. An X-ray showed a small abscess of the root filling material beyond the tooth apex. Extraction of the tooth and curretage of the area removed all symptoms.

STABBING THROAT/NECK PAIN

Two other cranial nerve neuralgias involve the *glossopharyngeal*, which supplies the tongue and the upper pharynx and the *greater occipital*, arising from the top of the cervical spine. They are described here by neurologist Robert Frank. The principles of treatment are similar to trigeminal neuralgia.

Glossopharyngeal neuralgia

The pain is usually located in the *lower part of the throat, the small area between the tonsils or at the base of the tongue.* The ear can also be involved. *The pain is described as stabbing, hot, shooting or electric.* The attacks are of short duration, lasting 20–30 seconds, interspersed with pain-free periods. Inciting influences may be swallowing, chewing or ingestion of liquids, cold or hot. Yawning, coughing, blowing the nose or extending the tongue may also incite the pain.

Greater occipital neuralgia

Here the area involved is the *entire posterior part of the scalp*, extending to the posterior borders of the ear. It is *almost always on one side and the pain is usually severe*. Generally it starts in the region of the neck and radiates upwards, but is sharp in onset, a twisting knife-like pain or electric shock. It may be limited to a single episode but generally volleys of shooting pain occur that end as abruptly as they begin. Certain actions can precipitate this pain, such as putting on a hat, combing the hair on the back part of the head or performing certain movements of the neck.

ATYPICAL FACIAL PAIN

Atypical facial pain, as its name implies, means pain that is not typical. There is no apparent cause and it is not, like trigeminal neuralgia, lancinating. It has been described as *a continuous dull ache with intermittent excruciating throbbing episodes located to a non-muscular site such as the jaw bone.* It is not provoked by jaw movements and rarely relieved by painkillers. Bouts of pain may last for hours or days.

Dr Charlotte Feinmann, pain specialist, writes: 'The pain mechanism appears to be vascular and the patient often suffers from other pains with a muscular or migrainous quality which may include neck, shoulder and back pain.' There may, however, be a link with trigeminal neuralgia, as Dr Feinmann explains.

> In some patients, a paroxysmal trigeminal neuralgia can provoke a more continuous atypical facial neuralgia, possibly due to a reactionary depression resulting from the primary neuralgia. The clinician may erroneously assume the neuralgia has become uncontrollable and requires surgery, whereas the therapy should include an antidepressant drug in addition to Tegretol. One also encounters the occasional case of trigeminal neuralgia which suddenly changes its character from an intermittent paroxysmal pain controlled by Tegretol to a more continuous pain responding only to antidepressant drugs.

JAW JOINT (TEMPROMANDIBULAR) PAIN

The tempro mandibular, or jaw joint, is the smallest joint in the body – and the one most exposed to the stress of movement as it opens and closes thousands of times a day. Problems with the joint are held to be responsible for a wide variety of different symptoms, varying from a *clicking, uncomfortable jaw joint on chewing, talking and yawning, to a continuous dull ache often described as earache*. The pain can radiate widely up into the skull and down into the jaw. There may also be associated symptoms such as headaches, disturbed hearing and tinnitus. The syndrome of tempromandibular dysfunction was first described back in 1934 by James B. Costen, who attributed it to poor occlusion, or malocclusion, of the upper and lower sets of teeth. This theory, however, is disputed. Dr Robert Frank observes:

> This disorder is treated in consultation with a dentist knowledgeable and interested in this field. The cause of the disorder is dental occlusive disease and treatment is generally directed towards improvement of the occlusion through various means. Physical methods of pain relief including heat, hot packs and massage are frequently employed and helpful.

NOCTURNAL JAW PAIN

Query Mrs P.J. from Gloucester, writing on behalf of her 77-year-old husband:

He has always been a healthy, active man till a few months ago when he started having *severe pain in his jaw. It almost invariably happens in bed in the early hours of the morning* and lasts 20–30 minutes. It leaves him feeling exhausted, with very tender gums. He also often gets a severe pain across his shoulders which comes on at lunch time – and necessitates him lying down for an hour or so. After exhaustive tests he had an angiogram in order to rule out angina, which it did.

Comment There was no satisfactory response to this query, though it would seem that jaw pain can be a feature of both acid indigestion and problems with the jaw joint.

(i) *Acid indigestion*: 'I too have been woken early by pain in the jaw extending downwards like toothache but diffuse and not traceable to a particular tooth. In my case it was due to indigestion, treatable by taking a couple of Rennies, repeated sometimes.'

(ii) *Jaw joint*: 'I also have this pain that affects the jaw and shoulders, with extremely sore gums. It is worse at night when the jaw is in one position for some hours – and I find I have to consciously "work" my jaw back to normal when it awakens me.'

MISCELLANEOUS FACIAL PAIN

The main categories of facial pain are described above, but every case is different and there are numerous variations of which here are a further two – the first due to spectacles and the second unexplained.

'Wind Blowing on my Cheek'

Query Mrs L.K. from Northampton writes:

Over several years I had an *annoying sensation in the right cheek – it was almost like constant wind blowing*. My doctor was sympathetic and sent me to various specialists where I had my sinuses inspected and surgery on the roots of my teeth (most inconvenient and uncomfortable). The condition continued! Eventually I was referred to a psychiatrist who prescribed valium! I enquired how long I would be taking this drug. 'For the rest of your life,' came the reply. I was then aged about 55. I graciously declined and ceased further appointments. At this stage I found a new optician and persuaded him to prescribe bifocal contact lenses for me. They were a huge success and my face problem ceased immediately! Now it only returns on the odd occasion when I revert to wearing glasses. The simple explanation was pressure on a nerve from my spectacles.

The Cricket Bat Sting

Query 74-year-old former estate agent Mr W.R. from Bristol writes:

> It started with a *sensation of tingling/burning in my upper right teeth and jawbone and some facial pains around my right upper cheek, also along the right edge of my tongue* – it only ever occurred on the right side of the face. When it is really bad I would describe it to people as like being hit on the side of the face with a cricket bat. The funny thing is I have never had these pains or sensations in bed and do not have any trouble sleeping. When I get up in the morning and start to move about I am aware of either a pain or sensation after about ten to 15 minutes. Sometimes it lasts for a few hours, sometimes all day, sometimes a few days or longer, but I seem to be always aware of it. There are a few things I find quite unable to explain. The most obvious is that when we are on holiday, in Scotland a few weeks ago, or in Spain for about two months in the winter, I very rarely get this pain.

Comment There were no suggestions as to the cause of this pain though, Mr W.R.'s own view is that 'it is some form of neurological malfunction – possibly stress related, but this must be subconscious stress as my life is fairly stress free!'

6
Vertigo and Collapse

The terms 'dizziness' and 'vertigo' are often used interchangeably, but there is actually quite an important distinction. Dizziness encompasses sensations such as feeling woozy, or disoriented or light headed, which if they occur, for example, on rising from a chair or on exertion, are usually due to a reduction of blood flow to the brain either from shock, low blood pressure or disturbance of heart rhythm. Vertigo, by contrast, is the more disturbing sensation, where the external world loses its stability, so the room and objects within it seem to be rotating or at a tilt. There are, as will be seen, many possible different causes for vertigo – but in one way or another, all involve a disturbance of the balance mechanism that allows us to stand upright without falling over and move our head from side to side while our visual perception of the world remains static.

This balance mechanism has three main components. The first is the middle ear, in particular the three semi-circular canals – or labyrinths – which are set at right angles to each other. They are filled with a fluid called lymph and come together in a common chamber, or vestibule. When the head tilts to right and left or back and forward, this lymph swishes around, brushing against minute hairs whose movement transmits nervous impulses indicating the position of the head and body at any given moment.

These messages are passed to the brain stem, which connects the brain to the spinal cord. Here they are coordinated with other sources of information on the position of the body from which it is forwarded to the brain, where the sense of position is perceived.

Vertigo may thus be a symptom of many problems to do with the ears, the brain stem or the brain itself. Most of the time there are other clues which point to the source of the mischief, so vertigo associated with tinnitus and loss of hearing is strongly suggestive of some problem with the inner ear. The focus here is rather on those situations where vertigo is the major or dominant symptom, and which can usefully be subdivided into the acute, recurrent and chronic.

ACUTE VERTIGO

Viral Infection

The sudden onset of acute vertigo is most often due to an acute viral infection of the middle ear, known as vestibular neuronitis (inflammation of the nerve arising from the 'vestibule' of the semi-circular canals). It can be very alarming, as the following account from a woman in her early 30s reveals:

> I woke that morning and lifted my head off the pillow only to be *overwhelmed by a sensation that the room was spinning around and around*. As I collapsed back on the bed, sweat pouring off my brow, *I realized I desperately needed to throw up*, but the bathroom seemed a million miles away. Very slowly I rolled onto my side, slid out of bed and crawled on my hands and knees towards the lavatory bowl. After a protracted bout of vomiting, I crawled back, phoned the doctor's surgery and managed to slip back into bed where I lay absolutely still.
>
> I thought I was dying and the only question was whether it was from a stroke, haemorrhage, brain tumour or heart attack. My doctor, however, was genuinely reassuring, pointing out that there are very few circumstances where such catastrophic symptoms actually turn out to be quite benign – but this apparently is one of them. I had an acute inflammation, probably caused by a virus, of the balance mechanism in my middle ear. A few days in bed, some pills to stop me feeling sick – and with luck all would be well.

Migraine

When the episodes of vertigo are similarly acute and occur several times a year, this is strongly suggestive of migraine.

Query Mr J.D. from Lincolnshire writes:

> I have had occasional spells of vertigo in the past but they generally lasted two or three days and, although unpleasant, did not greatly inconvenience me. *A few years ago I had a really severe attack which lasted for about two weeks and was initially accompanied by nausea. For a short period I even found it necessary to hold on to furniture in order to walk.* Since then I have had similar episodes at intervals of about nine months. I occasionally have the feeling that something is moving in the back of my head and on sitting up I feel as if I have a hangover without the headache.

Comment This type of migrainous vertigo can go undiagnosed – and therefore untreated – for years, as Dr Robert Baloh of the UCLA School of Medicine, Los Angeles describes:

> A 71-year-old woman reported recurrent dizziness over the past 50 years. Her episodes were characterized by a *'swimming sensation' in her head, along with nausea and vomiting, difficulty with concentration and a feeling of unsteadiness when attempting to walk.* During an attack she experienced a marked sensitivity to movement and preferred to lie completely still. Her dizzy spells typically lasted from 12–15 hours, but one had lasted as long as a week. The frequency was about once every three weeks. She also reported severe headaches every one or two years since her late 20s. Her maternal aunt had similarly recurrent dizziness and her son had migraine.

Approximately a quarter of migraine sufferers are afflicted by such episodes of vertigo, which can occur quite separarely from the usual headache. Most cases of benign recurrent vertigo in adults are caused by a migraine and patients often report migrainous headaches at other times in their lives. The mechanism is not well understood, but is probably due to spasm of the artery supplying the blood to the inner ear. It should respond to anti-migraine treatment.

RECURRENT VERTIGO

There are two main types of frequent episodes of vertigo which are less acute and shorter lasting (minutes rather than hours) than the migrainous variety just described.

Benign Paroxysmal Positional Vertigo (BPPV)

This type, as its name implies, is relatively mild and of short duration (benign), frequent (paroxysmal), and related to position (positional).

Query Mrs J.L., a translator from Bournemouth writes: '*I feel dizzy with sudden changes of position but not at any other time* – not when I am walking, for example. The condition seems to be occurring more frequently as I get older and the various medications I have tried have not worked.'

Comment This type of vertigo which occurs when moving the head is most probably due to the presence of small crystals of calcium in the semi-circular canals which brush against the hair-like projections sending false or distorted messages to the brain that are perceived as vertigo.

Treatment The treatment as recommended by ENT specialist John Epley from Oregon can best be described as analogous to the frustrating games so often given as Christmas presents, where the challenge is to shift small beads from one compartment to another in a closed glass box. Dr Epley devised a series of manoeuvres of the head by which the debris of calcium crystals is gently nudged out of the semi-circular canals into the roomier common chamber, or vestibule – and quite astonishingly it works.

The same principle presumably explains the 'miracle cure' of BPPV as described by Mr Leslie McDonald from Solihull while on a cruise in the Bay of Biscay. Mr McDonald's vertigo was brought on by sudden changes in position: 'When I brought my head down after looking up, when I laid my head on the pillow or rolled over in the night, the room would spin around for a few seconds.' After three months of this, he and his wife went on a cruise. 'The Bay of Biscay was a bit rough and many passengers were unwell. After a couple of days staggering about the decks, I found I no longer had vertigo and have been fine ever since.'

Spinal Vertigo

When vertigo is obviously related to movements of the neck or sleeping in one position, it may be that the cervical spine is pressing on the blood vessels supplying the balance mechanism in the brain stem.

Query 1 74-year-old retired school teacher Mr L.J. from Dorset writes:

I suffer from dizzy spells in my sleep. These only occur when I am sleeping on my left side, forcing me to turn over sharply to my right side. The dizziness then stops at once. This can happen from one to four times a night but not every night. Often weeks go by without anything happening. I never seem to suffer any dizzy spells when awake. I have had this for the last seven years.

Query 2 Mrs A.D. from Powys writes:

Some years ago I fell asleep on a longish journey with my neck on a 'blow up' horseshoe-shaped neck rest. I woke feeling my neck did not feel quite right. Later I went my doctor as *I was getting giddy when I bent to the left or slept on my left side.* I had an X-ray which showed that something had got misplaced in my neck which was pressing on the main artery to the brain. The doctor advised treatment at a sports centre injury clinic and told them 'no manipulation at all'. I went once a week for about four weeks and I lay on my front with a hole for my face downwards (very comfortable!) and had a heat lamp left warming the back of my neck. When the time was up with my neck nice and warm someone very gently finger-tipped stroked the back of my neck. My giddiness went and I have never had it since.

Dr G.M.S. Ryan reports a similar case:

A 57-year-old man had been in excellent health 'since a baby'.

While he was building a wall, a brick had struck him on the head; his neck was flexed at the time and the blow jarred his neck to one side. He felt 'sick and dizzy' for a few moments but was not unconscious nor did he fall. On recovery from the shock he noted *a severe pain across the back of the neck and up the back of the head, made worse by bending the head backwards and particularly on looking to the left*. He carried on with his work throughout the day and, apart from the pain, felt quite well. On lying down that night, however, he had a sudden and fairly severe attack of vertigo – 'everything started going round and I felt sick'. He did not vomit and after a minute or two the vertigo subsided. Over the following two weeks he noticed that on lying down or looking upwards with the neck extended he experienced intense, brief bouts of vertigo. These all gradually became less severe and by the time the pain had disappeared they were troublesome only on bending the head far back.

CHRONIC PERSISTENT VERTIGO

Those who are unfortunate enough to have persistent vertigo day in day out almost certainly have some chronic underlying condition which, in the ear, might be Meniere's disease or the inflammation of the semi-circular canals known as labyrinthitis; or in the brain, some persistent disturbance of function due to a stroke, or other inflammatory or degenerative process.

Query 1 82-year-old former headmaster Mr G.D. from Devon writes:

I have lived a very athletic life. My cricketing days finished when I was 50 and at 70 I was still dog walking miles each day. I then developed *almost perpetual dizziness, so that walking is a matter of clutching the furniture or pushing my wheeled walker*. When sitting bolt upright the symptom is less pronounced and this appears when I am lying flat.

Query 2 65-year-old former sailor from Weymouth, writes:

'*I suffer from vertigo when walking* and manoeuvring round the house has become an obstacle course to be tackled with military precision. In the prone position I feel fine, though my sleep pattern is undisturbed.'

Comment This form of chronic vertigo can be very difficult to evaluate and even more difficult to cope with. Every effort must be made to exclude some treatable underlying problem, such as a benign tumour of the auditory nerve (an acoustic neuroma) or benign hydrocephalus (increased fluid in the brain), as illustrated by the following account from Mrs M.E. from Leicester:

> My mother started to suffer dizzy spells – the doctor said vertigo. It worsened, the doctor said 'It's your age – vertigo.' I rang her one day to find her in tears. She was getting around the house with a shopping trolley in one hand and an upright vacuum cleaner in the other. Eventually I managed to get another doctor to come and see her and she was sent to hospital where, after various tests, it was found she had fluid on the brain. Her symptoms markedly improved following a lumbar puncture, but they came back. A permanent shunt was fitted to drain her excess spinal fluid away. From being homebound, she was able to return to a normal life.

Treatment Treatment is always difficult, though there is encouraging evidence that re-educating the brain to cope with the vertigo can be helpful. Ballroom dancers can twist and turn and gymnasts can do their exercises without feeling dizzy because the balance centre in the brain learns to adapt quickly to increased stress laid upon it. Similarly, those with chronic vertigo can gain relief by repeatedly inducing the sensation of dizziness, as described by Mrs M.B. from Lincolnshire:

> Some 30 years ago I had a *very bad attack of dizziness which for several days left me literally crawling along the floor.* After this I periodically suffered from dizzy attacks. I eventually saw a neurologist who told me the hairs in the ear which govern balance had been damaged. His advice was 'hold securely on to something. Tilt the head to one side and slightly back, wait for the dizziness to subside and do the same thing the other side. This "wears out" the balance mechanism for two–three hours, when the procedure can be repeated.

Finally, several readers describe how their vertigo improved with various alternative remedies:

(i) *Acupressure*: 'I first became aware of vertigo when sitting watching TV one Saturday three years ago. The room suddenly started to spin round and I could not stand up without the help of my husband, who managed with great difficulty to get me to the bathroom where I was violently sick. Next day my doctor called and said it could last three days or much longer – it has. Recently a friend who was going to Denmark by sea purchased from her chemist some wrist bands for seasickness, should I not try them? This I have done and although not cured, I really did not think they would benefit me. I do notice the difference if I leave them off. Now after three years and nine months I hardly notice the dizziness so long as I wear the wrist bands.'

(ii) *Gingko Biloba*: Gingko Biloba is a natural Chinese remedy from the Maiden Hair tree which reputedly lives an astonishing 4,000 years. It is reported to produce considerable improvement in several conditions related to the circulation and also in Meniere's disease. 'I have suffered from Meniere's and also deafness for many years. Ever since taking one Gingko Biloba tablet each morning the problem has disappeared! They are quite expensive but a small price to pay for such wonderful relief.'

(iii) *Vitamin E*: 'Nearly 16 years ago, at the age of 61, without any warning I had a violent attack of vertigo. I could not stand and every time I tried to straighten up I was dizzy and violently sick. My symptoms persisted until I read a book which recommended strong doses of Vitamin E. I took this advice and my attacks reduced from once a week to once a month and onwards, the gap increasing all the time. I now lead an active live, gardening, walking, ballroom dancing every week. It was interesting to find that the only deterioration I found was when I forgot to take my Vitamin E tablets on holiday abroad.'

(iv) *Temporomandibular Jaw Joint*: 'In 1968 I suddenly experienced earache in my right ear and suffered from loss of balance which made me feel quite ill. I had lots of tests including three days in hospital, and even wore a collar for some time. Nothing seemed to help and I still suffer from intermittent earache. Eventually I was referred to an oral specialist in Manchester who felt my problem may be due to damage to the temporomandibular joint following a slight prang in the car when I had had a very stiff neck for a few hours afterwards. He made a splint or bite riser which I had to wear night and day. It was like magic. I immediately started to improve. My balance slowly started to return to normal and the attacks of acute earache finally stopped. I have from time to time over the years suffered a slight recurrence of the balance problem, but I always resume wearing a splint and it gradually settles down again.

COLLAPSE ('DROP' ATTACKS)

There are, as can be imagined, many reasons why a person should suddenly collapse and fall to the ground, such as an epileptic fit, fainting or following a stroke. The concern here, though, is the more unusual situation where in the absence of such very obvious causes (and they usually are quite obvious), the person suddenly falls to the gound without loss of consciousness. These episodes are sometimes referred to as 'drop attacks', as the person literally drops to the floor. The explanation – especially in the older age group – is a temporary reduction of blood flow to the brain, either from a sudden fall in blood pressure (especially on rising) known as orthostatic hypotension, or a reflex slowing of the heart following movement of the head (carotid sinus syndrome). These are treatable with medication or, if necessary, a pacemaker.

Several other possibilities, however, must be considered.

Swallowing Syncopy

Query Mr B.E. from Harrogate writes on behalf of his 86-year-old wife:

> About *three times a week, immediately after breakfast* (cereal and one slice of wholemeal bread), *my wife collapses in a heap. I get her to bed and by lunchtime she is perfectly normal.* Her GP and consultant are totally baffled and cannot suggest any reason. Everyone here seems baffled. We cannot expect too much at our

age – but the unpredictability of what my wife calls 'floppiness' makes it difficult to plan anything such as a holiday.

Comment The unusual feature of this case is undoubtedly its close relationship to the first meal of the day, which raises the possibility of swallowing syncopy, where stimulation of the nerves in the wall of the oesophagus on swallowing induces a reflex slowing of the heart and subsequent reduced blood flow to the brain.

Dr Brian Olshansky from Illinois describes a similar case in a 72-year-old man who reported that carbonated drinks seemed to trigger several episodes of sudden collapse over a period of a year. After the most thorough investigations revealed nothing, he perhaps inadvisedly drank a can of Pepsi Cola while driving and wrecked his car. Dr Olshansky advised repeating the tests after drinking a can of Pepsi, at which point it became clear that his heart rate fell dramatically together with his blood pressure, thus accounting for his symptoms.

Mrs E.W. from Middlesex describes the same problem as it affected her:

> I am 86 and until two years ago suffered episodes of trembling and feeling weak. My GP was completely at a loss for a diagnosis, suspecting a heart condition, and had me on his couch on a number of occasions. Then I suffered a dental ulcer, requiring the removal of a tooth which had previously been crowned. This occasioned my going on a liquid diet for a few days. The significant fact was that I was completely relieved of my debilitating symptoms. Considering these always manifested in mid-morning, I suspected my breakfast of white bread, toast and marmalade. Following a change to cereal and bananas I was 'cured' except for occasions when I tried a cereal such as muesli which contained a powdery flour-like element.

Migrainous Syncopy

Migraine can cause drop attacks by producing spasm of the arteries to the brain, with subsequent reduction of blood flow. Dr James Lance of the University of New South Wales descsribes the following case:

A 40-year-old woman had a five-year history of drop attacks. *Each was preceded by a sense of fatigue and nausea lasting for five minutes and after she felt an epigastric (stomach) sensation rising to her head she toppled to the ground.* She recovered consciousness after 30 seconds, but the attack left her with a throbbing left-sided headache accompanied by nausea and vomiting which persisted for two or three days.

These migraine attacks should respond to anti-migraine treatment.

Cervical Spine

Athritis of the cervical spine in the neck can cause pressure on the blood vessels with reduced flow of blood to the brain. Mrs H.H. from East Sussex reports:

I am 80, normally very energetic but every week for the last year or two I am *overcome with morning collapse*. I have had many tests, thinking I was seriously ill, but now accept it is a positional problem which I can now usually avoid by trying to lie with my neck aligned as far as possible with the spine; the use of a feather pillow which can be pushed into position helps to meet this, but I can still get attacks every two to three weeks. These are on rising and wear off in the course of the morning.

Mr G.J. van Norel from the Netherlands reports how stabilizing the cervical spine can cure this type of drop attack.

A 79-year-old man had ten drop attacks over a three-year period, each lasting about a minute and accompanied by transient difficulty in speaking and dizziness but no loss of consciousness. He also had a few episodes of paraesthesiae (pins and needles) and after his latest fall sudden neck pain. Radiographs of the cervical spine showed displacement of the vertebra and following an operation he had no more drop attacks.

7
Throat and Voice

CHRONIC SORE THROAT

The sore throat accounts for 150,000 medical consultations a year, which works out at about four per family doctor per week – and its treatment costs the Health Service £22.5 million. Most of the time the culprit is a viral infection which will get better within a week or so, while the more severe and persistent are due to tonsillitis or glandular fever that respond to the appropriate treatment. But what if the symptoms persist?

Query 63-year-old retired translator, Mr D.E. from North London, writes:

> For the last three months I have been suffering from a chronic sore throat even though I am a non-smoker, non-drinker, non-singer and do not engage in excessive amounts of talking. The symptoms appeared virtually overnight and have been with me daily ever since. *It is a dry sore throat with occasional slight dry cough often accompanied by a burning sensation.* There is no inflammation or swelling of the glands, no lumps, no cold or flu symptoms, no congestion or expectoration, no loss of voice. When acute it produces an aching in the windpipe. The throat seems all right when I first wake up but within an hour of rising (during which time I will have started to speak and also eaten and swallowed) the symptoms start up again. The throat becomes irritated after but not during eating. Swallowing and talking also make it worse. I have been told by a leading specialist that it is nothing serious, that

there is nothing 'sinister' in the throat and that sooner or later the condition will get better. I have tried gargling with soluble aspirin, regular steam inhalations, lots of throat soothing honey and lemon, glycerine pastilles, warm drinks and soups. Even a complete absence of talking for a whole week! All to no avail.

Comment This syndrome is analogous to the chronic cough following an attack of viral bronchitis, where the symptoms persist even though the underlying cause has resolved. Presumably this is because the tissues are not yet healed and so it takes longer than usual to resolve. Two other possible explanations are chemical sensitivity and acid reflux.

Chemical Sensitivity

♦ *Ozone*: A chronic sore throat may be caused by extended use of equipment such as computers, printers or televisions which produce ozone as a bi-product. Ozone is amongst the most irritant and toxic of gases, an overdose of which causes damage to the airways. Sensitive people may be subject to coughs, dry airways, runny noses and shortness of breath. It might help to have a reasonable circulation of air in the room to help break down ozone to oxygen.

♦ *Cleaning sprays*: 'I had a chronic sore throat last year when I started using a new spray for cleaning worktops in the kitchen and the bath. The spray is so easily breathed in and I was anxious to find out why I couldn't sing the hymns at church! Then after just about losing my voice altogether I finally worked out what was causing the problem. Now I use the mousse type which directs the cleaner down onto the surface.'

♦ *Air pollution*: 'Several years ago I worked in Central London right by a very busy junction and in hot weather had the window open. I noticed that by the time I arrived home in the much less polluted Surrey I had what felt to be the beginnings of a burning sore throat. These symptoms invariably disappeared over the course of the evening or by the next morning.'

♦ *Toothpaste*: 'After years of broken nights, hundreds of "fishermen's friends" and many bottles of cough linctus and visits to the doctor, it suddenly dawned on me that the toothpaste I was using was the cause of my dry throat. I changed to a herbal toothpaste and made sure I rinsed teeth and gums very thoroughly and gargled a few times. Hey presto! Normal throat and no broken nights!'

♦ *Plant allergy*: 'I had a chronic sore throat for over a year which defied diagnosis including a most uncomfortable gastroscopy. Eventually I formed the view I had become allergic to something and moved a plant from the bedroom (I had always hated the blessed thing!). The symptoms cleared up quickly and although sadly we do not have flowers and plants in the house, it is worth it to be free of the problems.'

Acid Reflux

Mr Anthony Narula, ENT specialist at Leicester Royal Infirmary, writes: 'The association of coughing with a sore throat makes it extremely likely this man has silent gastro-oesophageal reflux.' Dr James Kaufman, director of the Centre for Voice Disorders in North Carolina, strongly recommends long-term treatment (i.e. up to six months) with drugs such as Gaviscon coupled with antacid therapy at full doses.

(i) 'The sore throat could be acid refluxing from the stomach. The answer is to raise the head of the bed six inches, not eat within an hour of going to bed and avoid spicy foods and cucumber. The acid suppressant drug Zantac at night might help.'

(ii) I had similar symptoms for many years, coming on when the head went back on the pillow at night – I used to take throat pastilles in the vain hope of relief. Eventually I found out it was nothing to do with the throat – but to acidity not being neutralized in the stomach and rising into the throat area. So it is the acidity which has to be tackled and I was prescribed Zantac and – more effective – Losec. One tablet each night controls the acidity and all has been well since for years.'

VOICE DISORDERS

The voice is 'the window of the soul' and the vocal chords through which it is transmitted are amongst the most hard-working of all the structures in the body, opening and closing as we talk and sing, thousands of times a day. A viral infection of the larynx – or indeed just too much talking – results in hoarseness. The solution is to rest the vocal chords by talking less, not singing in church, dripping honey down the back of the throat and eating raw eggs:

> I used to sing in the church choir as a teenager and was due to sing a major solo on Easter Sunday. The previous evening I went to a party and was up till the early hours, talking, reciting and telling stories. When I woke later that morning, I discovered I had completely lost my voice. My grandmother, a professional singer, suggested I crack a large egg into a cup and swallow it down whole (not beaten). This I did, albeit with some reluctance, and sure enough my voice returned and I sang my solo.

There are, of course, many other causes of hoarseness – which can usually be readily diagnosed by the ENT surgeon peering down the back of the throat with his special instruments, which may reveal signs of inflammation, warts or nodules on the vocal chords or something more sinister. But what if the vocal chords appear normal, as they do in the following three syndromes?

Voice Fatigue

Query Former illustrator 82-year-old Mr G.H. from Surrey writes:

> *Whilst speaking* at a meeting of friends and colleagues *without warning my throat became parched* and I was unable to continue. At the time I assumed this was due to the room temperature and lack of saliva but the condition continued. I was referred to a

specialist. I have had an endoscopy, chest X-ray and blood test, all of which have proved negative, and still the condition persists. In the morning my voice is normal, but as the day progresses so the quality of volume deteriorates presumably as the saliva dries. I have been accustomed to reading and singing in church, but this is no longer possible.

Comment There were two quite different explanations offered for this unusual problem – loss of saliva secretion or spasm of the vocal chord mechanism, though of course Mr G.H. may well have had both.

Dry throat

The first possibility is that the 'parched sensation' is responsible for the voice problem. This would then make it one of the group of syndromes due to lack of lubrication from inadequate salivary secretions that also includes dry nose and dry mouth, considered elsewhere.

Treatment The treatment is self-evident, as you should try to replace the reduced salivary secretions with some other form of lubrication.

(i) 'I have suffered from the same voice problem for a couple of years. I visited a consultant after several months who said it was probably a virus and would not go until the summer. It did improve but then returned with a vengeance, with prolonged conversation causing the glands on either side of my neck to ache. There is no pain in actually talking or swallowing, only the desperate desire to stop talking. Shouting or singing brings it on immediately. I am very involved on committees and still lecture occasionally and the only comfort I get is chewing sugar-free gum which was recommended by my local chemist. I have tried spraying with artificial saliva, which works but is more inconvenient than chewing gum.'
(ii) 'My interest in teaching certainly brought home to me the wisdom of teachers in the USA in enjoining pupils to 'pee

pale': in other words plenty of fluid intake; preferably water.'

(iii) 'As a young singing student some 50 years ago, I was taught to always carry a water bottle and take frequent sips to lubricate the working parts. I have insisted on the same practice with my own students in recent years. Dehydration can be a very common problem with teachers, politicians, publc speakers as well as actors and singers. If a plant wilts and the leaves droop it tells us it needs water. Not quite so easy to evaluate in human beings!'

An alternative approach is to reduce intake of tea and coffee which, being natural diuretics, promote the excretion of fluid in the kidneys and thus predispose to dehydration. Further suggestions include:

(iv) *Synthetic saliva*: 'A spray of synthetic saliva is useful but not always convenient to carry around. When doing the housework, gardening or singing in the church choir I find a piece of chewing gum keeps my mouth moist.'

(v) *Lemon juice*: 'My doctor suggests immediate application of a few drops of lemon juice on the tongue (or you can use a lemon juice squeezy plastic bottle). It works immediately like a charm.'

(vi) *Nigroid tablets*: 'The only remedy is to suck nigroid tablets (pellets of liquorice and menthol). I always carry a box and one sucked slowly brings relief. At night I sometimes wedge a pellet between my teeth before sleeping. These little things were known as 'choir boys' in my husband's youth, as they were the only permitted "suckers".'

(vii) *Peardrops*: 'I go nowhere for the past 20 years without peardrops (or similar) permanently in a container in the car or handbag. At home I found that a dash of thick honey does the trick.'

(viii) *Herbal hot toddy*: The following herbal remedy promotes salivation: 2 cinnamon sticks, 4 cloves, a squeeze of lemon or lime, 1 teaspoonful of honey, grated or sliced ginger to taste, whisky or brandy to taste.

Mr Peter Frost, a dentist from Guy's Hospital in London,

warns that 'Peardrops, lemon juice and sugar-containing sweets can all play havoc with the teeth. Sugar-free chewing gum is excellent and Salogen works very well.'

Spasm of the vocal chords

The second possible explanation for Mr G.H.'s symptoms is spasm of the vocal chords (or spasmodic dysphonia) – literally episodic difficulty in talking – of which two types are recognized. For most, the spasm occurs in the muscles that close the vocal chords and results in a strangled staccato voice. Alternatively when the muscles opening the vocal chords are involved this leads to a weak, husky, whispering voice. In both, as in Mr G.H.'s case the problem becomes worse the more the voice is used. The vocal chords appear normal on examination and for this reason this condition was in the past thought to be primarily psychological in origin. More recently, observing the movement of the vocal chords through a fibreoptic endoscope has revealed the spasms mentioned above, for which the probable explanation is some abnormality of the nerves that control speech.

Treatment

(i) *Botulinum toxin*: Treatment involves abolishing the spasm by paralysing the relevant muscles with an injection of botulinum toxin. The effect is seen in six days and usually lasts for two to four months. Approximately 90 per cent of patients have a satisfactory voice most of the time following the injection. Side-effects may include slight difficulty in swallowing, a weak cough and pain at the injection site.

There were, in addition, three further suggestions:

(ii) *Alexander Technique*: 'F.M. Alexander was an Australian actor at the end of the nineteenth century who suffered very similar symptoms. Doctors were of no help, but by observing himself in the mirror he discovered that when he spoke he pressed his head back, thereby compressing the spine and causing a lot of tension. By releasing the tension and improving his posture generally, he effected a complete cure. Some years ago I had to make an announcement to a large choir and I feared that what I had to say might not be popular. Though I was a teacher in a large independent school and I had plenty of experience in addressing large groups without difficulty, on this occasion my voice was less than reliable. Our shrewd conductor suggested a couple of days later that I might take some lessons in the Alexander Technique. I had the good fortune to be recommended to an intelligent and efficient Alexander teacher. The dysphonia was soon on the mend, but the rest of the teaching was of such value I continued with it until retirement forced me to move to another part of the country.'

(iii) *Acid reflux*: 'I had a similar problem and after various investigations nothing abnormal was found. There was some acid reflux and it was suggested that acid fumes might be causing some spasm of the throat. Accordingly the consultant suggested a month's treatment of Zantac – and all I can say is that after three weeks there was a definite improvement.'

(iv) *Steroid sprays*: 'I am an asthmatic and it appears that the years of inhaling the preventor steroid puffers without gargling and rinsing have been the cause of my dry throat and voice problems. I can no longer sing either, a great sadness. Only when I moved house and therefore changed my family doctor was I told to rinse and gargle.'

Whispering Speech

Query Mrs Q.J. from Hampshire writes on behalf of her niece that for the last two years she has '*lost the ability to speak other than in a whisper*'. She has seen a specialist, who told her there is no underlying physical problem to account for her symptoms.

Comment Mr John Cherry, ENT specialist from Blackburn, points out that problems with the vocal chords result in hoarseness or distortion of the voice – but never whispering. This, rather, is almost always due to a disorder of the manner of speaking and is particularly common among young girls. The treatment, which involves relearning normal speech, is given by a speech and language therapist, and, says Mr Cherry, 'I have never seen it fail.'

♦ 'When I found myself unable to speak "except in a strange whisper" for six months I was referred to a speech therapist. I learnt to breathe properly and did voice exercises when I was out walking. I was found, quite by chance, also to have an underactive thyroid, which may well have been a contributory factor. My voice is still apt to get husky, but I have returned to yoga classes and a relaxing group. I drink lots of water and am gradually increasing my doses of thyroxin.'

♦ There is a parallel – or rather opposite – condition where the voice is much too loud. Those with vocal loudness are often unaware of the problem. The major emphasis of therapy is the reduction of tension in the intrinsic laryngeal muscles. Humming, especially when soft and slightly breathy, usually induces more relaxed phonation with a decrease in vocal roughness.

'Rarely Says a Word' (Elective Mutism)

Query Mr T.B. from Portsmouth writes on behalf of his daughter.

My daughter is aged 21 and attends art college. At home she is cheerful, pleasant and usually busy with her art activities. *Outside of the home she rarely says a word to anybody and has no friends or acquaintances.* Myself, my wife and my son are the only people she feels at ease with. With all other relatives, including her grandparents, she will only speak quietly and hesitantly after a good deal of prompting. She has seen a child psychologist who thought a particular event might be responsible. It all seemed a bit vague and produced no results. She could be called an 'elective mute' but there is nothing elective about it. In her words 'the harder I try to speak, the worse it is.'

Comment The term 'elective mutism' emphasizes the point that there is no underlying physical explanation for the difficulty in speech – thus the person can be presumed to have 'chosen', or 'elected' not to speak. It usually occurs in young children from the age of three or four onwards and is probably induced by the anxiety associated with excessive shyness or social phobia. Dr Paul Joseph of the New York University School of Medicine describes another case:

> A.L. is a four-year-old girl who has spoken no words to her teachers or classmates in the one and a half years she has been at school – despite speaking actively and well at home. There is no separational problem in sending her to school. She is not considered to be oppositional. She has no significant psychological problems and there is no known physical or emotional trauma before her entrance to school. Her mother considers her to be extremely shy. It is of particular interest that her mother did not speak in school until her high school years. Both parents have moderate anxiety in social situations. There is evidence that the drug fluoxetine can be helpful in some cases.

8
The Chest

There is a lot going on in the chest, with the heart, lungs and oesophagus all in close proximity, enclosed by the bones and muscles of the rib cage. The scope of symptoms to which they can give rise is legion and it is usually not difficult to determine what the problem is – but as will be seen, sometimes it can be!

SEVERE CHEST PAIN OF UNKNOWN CAUSE

Query 1 Mrs S., a 38-year-old housewife from Salisbury, writes:

> For most of my adult life I have suffered from *searing pains across my chest wall and under my armpits*. I have no warning of when this is going to occur and it is not triggered by any particular movements. The episode of pain can last from an hour or two or can punctuate the whole day. They vary in magnitude from appallingly intense – for which I seek relief with codeine – to the mildly uncomfortable, where the left arm itself seems to ache from shoulder to elbow. I tend to experience bouts of pain over a week or so and then apart from the odd mild sensation I may be essentially pain free for several months. I have consulted various doctors over the years but they seem to be unable to make any sense of my pain. Anything seriously wrong of a neurological nature has been ruled out – but nothing has been 'ruled in'.

Query 2 Mrs A.M. from Oxford writes on behalf of her 60-year-old sister-in-law who has suffered for a number of

years with pains in her chest for which no cause can be
found.

The pain can start at any time and can last from one or two days,
to five or more. It starts with *stabbing pains in the left back side
of the chest which move to the front centre of the chest, with sharp
stabbing pains in the front upper right of the chest.* The pains are
so severe that they make her catch her breath. At the same time,
she experiences *pains going up both sides of the neck behind the
ears and into her head.* During these episodes she feels extremely
ill, cannot remain in bed if it occurs during the night and 'doesn't
know what to do with herself' whenever they happen. All medical
avenues seem to have been explored and the specialist cannot find
an answer – but the problem continues causing her considerable
stress and anxiety with all helplines exhausted.

Comment The source of chest pain is usually quite clear-cut,
as the type of symptoms complained of are so specific: those
from the heart being 'tight', radiating down the arm and
brought on by exertion; from the lungs being sharp and stabbing and brought on by breathing and coughing; and from the
oesophagus, burning or heartburn made worse by leaning over
or lying down. The above chest pains clearly fall into none of
these categories – and so must be presumed to be arising from
the bones and muscles of the chest wall or the nerves that
supply them.

Chronic 'Lock Strain' on the Spinal Joints

Commenting on Mrs A.M.'s stabbing chest pains, osteopathic
physician Dr Tony Platts writes:

I suspect the sufferer has a form of chronic 'lock strain' (for want
of a better term) affecting one or other of the joints of the upper
dorsal spine. It is well recognized that one of these joints causes
pain (often referred) which is worse on movements affecting the
particular level of the spine and with associated restriction of
movement. After three to five days the symptoms and the strain
settle, but unless treated the locking persists. After varying intervals any repeated trauma to the affected joint, often only minor,

will call a restrain and recurrence of the pain. This is often enough reason to seek manipulation in the first instance.

The level of involvement in this case is likely to be the fourth thoracic vertebra (the 'T4 syndrome') which is one which is associated with symptoms that can affect the head, arm and hand around the chest and into the exilla.

Two further types of muscular chest pain are worthy of note:

Chest Wall Twinge Syndrome

Dr Adele Farm of the University of Toronto writes:

This is a rare, benign disorder of unknown cause characterized by episodes of very brief sharp anterior chest pain. It occurs in young healthy individuals usually near the tip of the heart. Some report the onset while *assuming a slouching or bent-over posture*. The pains last from 30 seconds to three minutes. They are aggravated by deep breathing and usually relieved by shallow respiration or assuming the correct posture.

Inflammation of the Rib Joint (Tietze's Syndrome)

Dr Gerald Levy from the Medical Center, Jersey City describes the following case history:

A 48-year-old white married salesman came to the outpatient clinic with *intermittent pain and swelling of four years' duration in the upper costosternal (where the ribs join the sternum) area*. The pain occurred both at rest and during exertion and was not related to time of day, lasting from several minutes to hours and occasionally lasting for days. Relief could be obtained by aspirin and the local application of hot compresses. Pain and swelling were limited to the left side initially and subsequently the right. Attacks occurred initially every few weeks and subsequently several times a week. Physical examination was unremarkable except for tenderness to palpation. He was initially treated with aspirin and told to apply hot compresses when necessary. Subsequently a monthly trial of steroids abated his symptoms. The cause of Tietze's syndrome remains unknown. It is especially important that patients be reassured of the benign character of the disorder.

ATYPICAL HEART PAIN (ANGINA)

The symptoms of angina due to narrowing of the coronary arteries are probably the best known of any serious illness, where – on exertion – a heavy pain grips the chest and radiates up into the neck and down into the arms. The following cases emphasize the importance of considering angina as a possible diagnosis for *any* symptom brought on by exertion – even in the absence of chest pain.

Headache

Dr Gaetano Lanza from Rome describes the following case:

A 68-year-old man was admitted with a three-year history of *brief episodes of headache at the back of the skull* which had been attributed to arthritis of the cervical spine. In the week before his admission his frequency of headaches had increased. While in hospital the patient had a two-hour headache with pain radiating from his shoulders. A routine laboratory test suggested a mild heart attack. The exercise test had to be terminated because the patient reported a typical headache. He underwent coronary artery bypass and has been free of symptoms and headaches in the three-year follow up.

Earache

Dr M. Morten Bryhn from Sweden reports the following case:

For several years a 67-year-old man had complained of *intermittent pain in the left ear initially described as a feeling of pressure*. Ear and nose examination was normal. Subsequently the ear pain became incapacitating. It was provoked by cold weather, physical exertion and emotion and was relieved after a brief rest. When the pain was excruciating it spread towards the shoulders and upper arm. Since the provocative factors were similar to those frequently encountered in angina, he was referred for cardio-vascular evaluation. An exercise test indicated reduced working capacity due to recurrence of the severe ear pain. He was considered for coronary bypass and coronary angiography revealed narrowing of the main coronary artery. Three weeks later while waiting for his operation he died suddenly from a heart attack.

Itching Nose

Dr Robert Reichstein of the Mount Sinai Hospital in New York reports the following case:

A 60-year-old man sought medical attention for *itching of the bridge of his nose*. The itching was associated with walking and sexual intercourse and was relieved by rest. Initial therapy consisted of mild analgesics and reassurance, but persistence of the nasal itching along with the development of shoulder pain prompted a return visit to the physician. An exercise tolerance test reproduced the nasal itching and after coronary angiography coronary artery bypass surgery was performed. In the nine months of follow up, there has been no recurrence of the itching.

PERSISTENT COUGH

The purpose of coughing, obviously enough, is to dislodge some irritant from the airways such as the inflammatory cells associated with a viral infection. Those whose cough lasts more than a few days will sooner or later have a chest X-ray, which may reveal a 'patch' of pneumonia or small tumour. The difficulty arises in trying to find out what is amiss in those whose cough persists even though their X-ray is normal – and here are several possibilities.

Upper Respiratory Tract Infection

Some of those with a long history of dry cough report that it followed an acute infection of the respiratory tract but, instead of getting better as usually happens within a few days, the cough has persisted for months or even years. Careful examination of the lining of the airways reveals some chronic damage which may allow irritants to penetrate more readily.

Treatment with steroids, either orally or inhaled, may be effective.

Post-Nasal Drip

Excess fluid produced by the lining of the nose (see Chapter 2, Runny Nose) can drip down the back of the throat into the lungs to cause a persistent dry cough, especially in the morning. Appropriate treatment is considered in the relevant section.

Asthma

A chronic cough, even without a wheeze, may be the only symptom of asthma, especially if it keeps children awake at night or follows exercise. Possible precipitating factors should be identified and anti-asthma medication is usually curative.

Acid Reflux

Reflux of the acidic secretions of the stomach may, besides causing heartburn, tip over into the airways to irritate the lungs – as described by Dr Paul Glasziou in a patient who had a chronic cough for over 20 years:

> Mrs V was a 66-year-old woman who said she had had a *non-productive cough daily* for 20 years. This had been treated unsuccessfully in the past with antibiotics, and anti-asthma medication. She was a non-smoker and had never lived with smokers. She did, however, report some heartburn, and so hoping to reduce the acid reflux I suggested as a simple first measure that she raised the head of her bed 10–15 centimetres and take 20ml of magnesium and aluminium hydroxide antacid at night. The cough settled within a few days and six months later had not returned.

Side-Effect of Drugs

The group of drugs known as Ace Inhibitors used for the control of raised blood pressure can cause chronic cough, as the following account by Nobel Prize winner Sir John Vane describes for reasons that will be obvious:

I have always been a strong supporter of Ace Inhibitors for treating hypertension, which is not surprising for I helped to invent them. I have been taking them myself for several years and one of those unfortunate who cough so much so that taking my once-a-day preparation in the morning sometimes led to retching. I am also prone to seasonal hay fever with itchy and runny eyes. My cardiologist reluctantly agreed to change my medication. Within the first six weeks of taking the new treatment, there was a dramatic reduction, not only in the cough but also in the eye and nose symptoms as well.

Large Tonsils and Elongated Uvula

Large tonsils at the back of the throat or an enlarged uvula (the fleshy part of the palate) can cause a chronic cough – as Dr Frank Miller from Cleveland describes in the following case:

> An 18-year-old male was referred for evaluation of *repeated episodes of dry cough and choking*. Physical examination revealed a healthy appearing man with a normal voice. But examination revealed an extremely elongated uvula. The patient was taken to the operating room and the uvula removed under general anaesthesia. He had an uneventful recovery and there has been no recurrence of the cough one year after the procedure.

Vagus Nerve Irritation

The vagus nerve is the longest in the body, running from the back of the brain down through the ear into the chest – where it helps control the heart rate – all the way down to the diaphragm. It may be involved in a chronic cough, as described in the following two cases.

♦ ENT surgeon Mr K.O. Poulose reports: 'A case was referred to us by our colleagues after they were unable to find a cause for a middle-aged patient's cough, in spite of extensive investigation. While examining his ears it was remarkable to find a few implanted hairs on the skin of the posterior canal touching the ear drum. On further questioning he was found to be an obsessive "self-ear cleaner". After removal of the hairs his symptoms disappeared. A similar dry cough associated with stimulation of the vagus nerve has been reported in association with impacted wax or a foreign body in the outer ear.

♦ Mr Majed Odeh of the Zion Medical Centre in Israel writes: 'A 74-year-old man was referred by his family physician for a cough he had had for 15 years. He was disturbed and despairing because despite extensive investigations no cause had been found. The previous year the episodes had become much more frequent, lasted longer and occurred almost every day and also at night. Physical examination was normal except for frequent dry coughs and an irregular pulse. While we were feeling the patient's pulse we noticed his cough always occurred when his pulse missed a beat, which an ECG showed was due to premature contraction of the atrium of the heart (atrial premature complex). This was treated with beta-blockers, the heart rate returned to normal and attacks of coughing decreased from many times daily to no more than a couple of episodes a week lasting only a few seconds.'

POUNDING HEART

Query A 70-year-old retired model, Mrs P.E. from Croydon, writes:

I find that when in bed, *my heart while beating at a regular rate, pounds in my chest and ears, which makes it difficult to get to sleep.* On waking the following morning there is a turbulence or quivering in the chest which extends down my arms to my fingers. On touching anything it feels as if it is moving. The symptoms dissipate as soon as I get up and move about.

Comment This pounding heart is generally considered to be evidence of overactivity of the nerves involved in controlling the activity of the blood vessels and organs – the autonomic nervous system – whose stimulation is often associated with symptoms such as pounding chest, trembling, sweating and hunger. It occurs in those with diabetes whose blood sugar has fallen too low (hypoglycaemia); as a feature of panic attacks; and as a symptom of over-use of the nitrate group of drugs, used in the treatment of angina.

It must be presumed the source of this mystery syndrome is similarly be related to over-activity of the autonomic nerves – but two other possible causes first have to be considered.

♦ *Heart rhythm abnormality*: If a pounding pulse, either too rapid or too regular, occurs at other times of the day and starts and stops abruptly, this is strongly suggestive that there is some intermittent abnormality of heart rhythm. A reader from Cheshire writes: 'I was diagnosed with a heart flutter, the symptoms of which include both excessive sweats, more pronounced when in bed, and a pounding of the heart on going to bed, which increased when I lay on my left side. I experienced what could best be described as a bubbling feeling in the chest which cleared soon after I got up and moved about, but the fast heartbeat continued. Appropriate medication has brought matters back to normal.'

♦ *Pulsatile tinnitus*: When the pounding chest is 'heard' in the ear as an auditory sensation like tinnitus, there is a possibility there may be some abnormality of blood flow in the vicinity. This can often be detected by listening over the ear with a stethoscope. There are a range of possible diagnoses and an ENT specialist should be consulted.

Treatment The following suggestions were received for the lady from Cheshire's pounding heart but there were no comments on her associated 'vibrations'.

(i) *Wax*: 'I have also experienced something very similar together with a slight feeling of nausea similar to the mild discomfort of sea sickness. The feeling of imbalance gave me the clue to these symptoms, so I visited my doctor for an ear examination which confirmed I had a very considerable build up of wax in both ears – although at no time had I been

conscious of a deterioration in my hearing. Subsequent syring-
ing and removal of the wax resulted in an instant return to
normality with complete cessation of the syndrome.'

(ii) *Raise the bedhead*: 'I experienced symptoms described to a
lesser degree, if I have to sleep in a bed where the head is even
half an inch lower than the foot. This sometimes happens in
old houses where the floors are uneven. One extra pillow
makes no difference, but something under the legs of the head
of the bed to raise it just slightly works instantly.'

(iii) *Caffeine*: 'I have experienced a pounding in my chest and
ears at night which makes it difficult to get to sleep, and this
seems to be associated with drinking too much coffee too late
at night. If I am careful what I drink before going to bed the
pounding of my heart does not happen.'

The association with 'trembling' seems to be unresolved – but
two other readers described similar symptoms:

♦ 'About two or three times a week *I wake with my lower
torso quivering* and trembling, I can feel this not only
inside but when I put my hands on my body.'

♦ 'I notice *as I leant on the breakfast table I could feel a
slight tremble in my arm* although no trembling was
visible. Over a period of weeks the feeling of trembling
seemed to have spread to my stomach and chest area,
sometimes waking me in the night with a feeling of a
rapid heartbeat. The trembling was hardly noticeable
during the day, but could be felt at rest especially in bed
at night.

INVOLUNTARY INSPIRATION

Query Mrs H.A. from Surrey writes: 'When I am at rest in bed
or sitting down quietly, I am obliged to take *a short sharp
involuntary breath* for no particular reason and at random. I
have had this condition for two years.'

Comment This involuntary inspiration is variously described as a 'silent hiccup' or a 'pulmonary yawn'. It would appear to be quite common, but has never properly been described before. Three possible explanations were suggested.

Lack of Oxygen

'I have always thought this an entirely normal physiological response to compressing the lungs by sitting in a slumped or semi-recumbent position in an armchair or sofa. Eventually one is just getting insufficient oxygen and the diaphragm contracts to force air in.'

Sleep-Related Reflex

It is well recognized that jerks and other sudden movements occur just prior to sleep and this involuntary inspiration may be a variant of this.

- 'I experienced the symptoms at times of relaxation principally in the twilight zone between wakefulness and sleep, when a sudden fierce involuntary intake of breath renders me instantly awake. I have long since assumed the condition poses no real threat and is rarely embarrassing as it occurs mostly in private and appears not too progressive.'
- 'I have experienced this odd affliction – a sort of involuntary jerk – for two or three years now. It affects me when lying down, usually preparatory to sleep.'

Heart-Related Reflex

Involuntary inspiration can be associated with abnormalities of heart rhythm.

- 'I was forced to retire early at the age of 59 because of irregular heart fibrillation, the symptoms of which began in just the same way as described. In my case I breathe through my mouth so the "short sharp involuntary breath" took the form of a single hiccup. I realized something was wrong when these could be heard in a crowded room!'

♦ 'I understand it is a result of the heart reasserting its normal rhythm when it has been irregular. It happens only when I am sitting and I am aware of it only as it happens, not before.'

♦ 'I have had this curious phenomenon over several years. Mine dates from having a cardiac pacemaker fitted. I have met another pacemaker recipient with the same manifestation.'

EXCESSIVE YAWNING

Query A 76-year-old retired SRN, Mrs J.M. from Cambridge, writes: 'I am troubled by *long bouts of yawning at any time of day* and even in town when shopping or out walking the dog, or when driving. Sometimes I feel drowsy at intervals but mostly I just feel very tired for minutes on end. Then the symptoms disappear for varying lengths of time.'

Comment Yawning when tired – which is more frequently associated with stretching – is an attempt to regain, albeit only temporarily, a state of alertness. It was originally thought that yawning was intended by nature to be 'a gymnastic . . . an automatic impulse caused by bad air in the lungs which awakens the respiratory organs into activity'. It might seem plausible that the large intake of air that accompanies the initial yawning and respiratory effort might boost the oxygen supply to the brain. This, however, has been discounted in the absence of evidence that tiredness is due to oxygen deficiency. More recently it has been suggested that stretching of the arms and respiratory muscles is the crucial factor, revitalizing the body by counteracting the loss of muscle tone that comes with tiredness.

Protracted yawning may indicate the incapacitating but

treatable condition known as Primary Disorder of Vigilance where those affected find it difficult to concentrate and stay awake. Dr Warren Weinburg of the University of Texas describes the case of a nine-year-old boy whose teachers thought he was lazy and immature: 'He yawned a lot, and was easily bored. He disliked reading and was unable to concentrate on any task.' Dr Weinburg treated him with amphetamine-like stimulants 'with immediate improvement ... he read 59 books in four months and built a model of the Hoover dam out of 25,000 toothpicks'. This primary disorder of vigilance is distinguished from other causes of excess sleepiness such as narcolepsy because it tends to run in families. The children affected have a quite characteristic temperament – usually described as being kind, caring and compassionate.

Excessive yawning has also been described as a side-effect of treatment with the anti-epileptic drug Epilim and in association with periodic limb movements in sleep, which is treatable with the anti-Parkinson's Levodopa.

None of these explanations, however, apply to this case, for which the following suggestions have been made:

Allergy

♦ 'I would suggest the bouts of yawning and tiredness may be due to an allergy. I have managed to avoid these symptoms of many years by cutting out all wheat, rye, barley and oatmeal from my diet.'

♦ 'For many years I would feel exhausted almost though I were drugged, I had to force myself to keep going, yawning, and could hardly keep my eyes open. Then after an interval I would suddenly snap out of it and feel normal again; as quickly and suddenly as switching off a tap. My life has been revolutionised since discovering that I am extremely intolerant of dairy products. I have now cut right back on them with the result that I am wide awake, raring to go and with more energy at 62 than 22.'

Neck Injury

♦ 'Over 20 years ago I was in a nasty car accident and sustained a whiplash, which broke the neck of my first left rib. Ever since then, if I put my head back to look at something high up, I invariably start a spell of deep yawning – I try to remember never to look up, but inevitably I sometimes forget. If sightseeing, perhaps in a cathedral, I have to ask my husband to stand behind me supporting my neck, so I can lean back rigid to look at the roof. Alternatively I lie flat on the floor. At the time of my accident my GP had a similar one. He too experienced yawning spells if he put his head back. We theorized this was due to our broken bones that when moved backwards pressed on the vagus nerve and that this triggered off the yawning. Incidentally when travelling by car in mountainous country with a series of U bends I put on my stiff medical collar – if I don't I soon start to yawn.'

♦ 'I too have bouts of yawning which can go on and on. Five years ago I broke my neck in a sailing accident. I have had a metal plate inserted and don't have much flexibility in looking up or down. A number of times my husband has remarked on it and said it "can't be normal".'

WRIGGLING DIAPHRAGM

Query Mr B.B. from Berkshire writes on behalf of his 55-year-old wife: 'My wife has experienced a *'wriggling sensation' in her diaphragm* which she can only liken to the movements of a baby in the womb. Investigations have found nothing wrong.'

Comment I am unable to identify any previous description of this syndrome which elicited the following four very different explanations:

Muscle Spasm

Over some weeks the sensation intensified until it actually became possible for my husband and I clearly to see the diaphragm area 'jumping'. Having seen *Alien* I began to entertain some ridiculous thoughts! At the time I was attending a clinic for back pain and the practitioner said this could be strong intermittent muscle spasm. He explained that localized pressure on the muscle might correct this, but warned it would be 'hard to take'. I lay down and then with his hand only he applied pressure with such strength and weight I could only just bear it and gasped in the very shallowest of breaths. Pressure was maintained for possibly 30 seconds or more. That was 12 years ago and from that day the problem never recurred.

Carbonated Drinks

I wonder if this lady is partial to carbonated drinks. I have suffered for years with a similar problem which could be quite alarming when it woke me at night. I mentioned it to my family doctor who said it could be caused by the gases staying in the stomach and rising up in my oesophagus at night when horizontal. Since giving up carbonated drinks the problem has gone.

Temporal Lobe Epilepsy

I experienced a similar feeling for several years and eventually suffered a short loss of consciousness, after which temporal lobe epilepsy was diagnosed. The same feeling in my abdomen, along with other symptoms, has always remained the early warning of an epileptic seizure.

Underactive Thyroid

I had my thyroid out to remove a tumour (which fortunately turned out to be benign). Shortly thereafter I began to suffer signs of an underactive thyroid: constant feeling of being cold, unable to get warm, putting on weight, lacking energy, and difficulty holding concentration whilst problem solving, and perhaps most noticeably, an odd sensation in the muscles around the diaphragm and lower abdomen. I would describe it as a crawling sensation. At its worst, it stopped me dead in my tracks with short duration muscle spasm. I have since settled at a daily dose of thyroxin. It isn't perfect but seems to work most of the time. If the dose is a little low I get a crawling sensation in the right side of my abdomen below the diaphragm, which although completely painless is uncomfortable – although nothing like as bad as before I was prescribed the thyroxin.

9
The Gut

The internal lining of the gut can now be scrutinized from 'top to toe' all the way from the back of the mouth down to the anus, thus revealing the common causes of bowel disorders – infection, inflammation, ulcers and so on – that were previously hidden from view. There is usually not much difficulty in knowing what to do to put things right. This seems quite straightforward, but is associated with a curious paradox, exemplified by the mystery syndromes considered in this section – that not infrequently nothing can be found to account for the patient's synmptoms. Thus those with difficulty in swallowing have normal oesophaguses, with ulcer pain have no ulcers, with nausea have normal stomachs and so on. These patients are then caught in the invidious situation of being told that 'everything seems fine' – with the obvious implication that their symptoms are 'psychological' – when they know only too well they are not.

And indeed their guts are not 'normal', nor are their symptoms, rather over the last ten years it has become apparent that the problem lies in the 'function' of the gut – how it propels its contents forwards or how the nerves in its lining perceive what is happening. Irritable Bowel Syndrome is the best known of these functional gut disorders but, as will be seen, they can occur in any part of the intestinal tract.

INTERMITTENT PAIN ON SWALLOWING

Query 1 56-year-old vet Mrs L.T. from Yorkshire writes:

For the last two years I have had intermittent episodes of severe pain at the base of my throat – sometimes nothing for a few days, sometimes waking me up several times in one night – which comes on very suddenly, spreads down into my chest and up into my jaw and is accompanied by salivation. I eventually discovered I could avert a full-blown attack by drinking as soon as possible.

Query 2 Mr D.W. from Huddersfield writes:

For the past 15 years I have been woken by a pain and have to walk the floor and sip hot water. It isn't possible to sit or lie down as that makes it even worse. It takes more than two hours to go away and allow me to go back to bed. At its worst it feels like a knife being stuck into the base of my gullet and the pain radiated in waves around my shoulder blades and into the back of my head. Part of the trouble is I salivate more so I have to go to the bathroom and spit it out rather than swallow.

Query 3 Mr P.H. from Yorkshire writes:

My problem occurs infrequently – but causes me considerable distress and embarrassment. It has happened about half a dozen times altogether, always when I have been dining in a restaurant. *When the meal is placed in front of me I eat the first two or three mouthfuls but then my digestive system seizes up.* I suddenly find I cannot eat or drink and my mouth fills with saliva. I do not get any pain unless I try to swallow. I then have to retire to the loo. The only solution seems to be to make myself vomit and then to try to get rid of the pocket of air which seems to be trapped under the food. This process takes the greatest part of half an hour. The whole incident is very distressing as afterwards I have to apologize to the restaurant management for not being able to eat their food.

Query 4 Mr E.J. from Kent writes:

I have three different but apparently related symptoms which occur at different times as follows:

I get a *pain behind the breastbone which spreads up to the underside of the jaw or throat.* This will slowly subside in up to ten minutes but is eased by sipping hot water, often accompanied by burping. This can happen at any time and is not connected with the intake of food or drink, such as during the night. Alternatively while eating food or drink it appears to come to a stop behind the breastbone *as if there was a blockage, accompanied by hoarseness and some difficulty in speaking*. This subsides after a minute or two, usually with some burping. This is uncomfortable rather than painful and usually happens only once during a meal, but not at every meal. It is more likely to happen at breakfast.

My third symptom occurs sometimes when drinking and consists of a *continuous minor bubbling or burping and regurgitation*. The first time it happened quite unexpectedly while drinking tea and was accompanied by violent regurgitation and spluttering. There was no pain or discomfort.

Comment There can, of course, be many possible reasons for pain and difficulty in swallowing – a hiatus hernia, strictures or a tumour – but when, as in these cases, the symptoms are intermittent and the lining of the oesophagus appears normal, it is possible to infer that the problem is due to episodic spasm of the surrounding muscles. The excess saliva is known as waterbrash, which will be considered below.

Treatment These episodes come out of the blue, though they can be precipitated by food and in particular very hot or cold drinks. The following treatments have been suggested:

(i) *Schnapps*: David Taylor, former Professor of Medicinal Chemistry at Belfast University reports: 'Oesophageal spasm completely prevents anything going up or down. It can last for some time and is very distressing. It can be completely and immediately fixed by a tot of Schnapps. Vodka is very good, but I imagine that any sort would do. Compared with the treatment, or lack of it, handed out by the medical profession, this ranks as a wonder of the world.'

(ii) *Peppermint*: 'I have suffered for years from extremely painful oesophageal spasm and can report an infallible cure, which is an extra strong peppermint. Relief is instant and lasting. Occasionally with a very bad attack I have taken a second, but only infrequently.'

(iii) *Drugs*: The drug GTN, used for the alleviation of anginal pains from the heart, can also abort an attack of oesophageal spasm. This can be very misleading, for the obvious reason that if the pain is falsely attributed as being due to angina, its relief by GTN appears to confirm the misdiagnosis.

(iv) *Nifedipine and other calcium blockers*: Dr Salah Nasrallah from Maryland writes: 'A 55-year-old man had a two-year history of difficulty in swallowing and a choking sensation upon swallowing liquid or solid food. The sensation lasted for three to five minutes and was not associated with pain or heartburn. He did not have any nausea, vomiting or weight loss. He was put on Nifedipine 10mg half an hour before meals and when re-evaluated four weeks after therapy the difficulty in swallowing and choking sensation had disappeared and he could eat without difficulty.'

(v) *Acid suppressant drugs*: In some patients, the trigger to the spasm is reflux of acid in the lower part of the oesophagus, in which case acid-suppressive medication should be effective. 'Two or three years ago I started to experience difficulty in getting food down, particularly at breakfast. Bread seemed to form a lump and lodge painfully in my oesophagus. This got steadily worse so I consulted our excellent GP, who sent me for a barium swallow. The findings were all negative. He then suggested I might try Lansoprazole, although I was never troubled by acid reflux. I have been taking this for about a year now with no adverse effect but complete resolution of my swallowing problem, as long as I remember to take a tablet first thing in the morning.'

(vi) *Surgery*: Approximately one in five patients with diffuse spasm may benefit from dilatation of the lower oseophagus. In those whose symptoms persist, then the definitive surgical procedure is an oesophagomyotomy (horizontal incision of the muscles around the oesophagus).

WATERBRASH

The production of excess saliva, as noted above, may be a dominant symptom of oesophageal spasm. When it occurs it is known as waterbrash, which is also believed to be related to acid reflux.

Query Mrs M.L. from Kirkudbrightshire writes: 'Without any notice, my stomach suddenly goes into spasm. *I feel as if I am going to be violently sick*, become dizzy and saliva shoots into my mouth. This lasts for two or three minutes before subsiding and happens several times a day every six months or so.'

Comment Waterbrash is an uncommon and frequently misunderstood symptom that applies to the sudden filling of the mouth with clear, slightly salty fluid. This fluid is not regurgitated material, but rather secretions from the salivary glands as part of a protective reflex when acid refluxes up into the lower oesophagus.

Dr Alan Birch, writing in the *Practitioners' Handbook*, observes: 'Waterbrash means a sudden appearance in the mouth of copious amounts of saliva which passes down the oesophagus and collects above the sphincter separating it from the stomach. Then, without nausea or a proper act of vomiting, it is shot up into the mouth and either spat out or swallowed.'

Treatment

(i) *Acid-suppressant therapy*: The trigger for the waterbrash being acid reflux, the obvious approach is to reduce the quantities of acid secreted by the stomach.

> For the past few years I have experienced a violent – really violent – upheaval in my midriff, immediately followed by saliva shooting into my mouth. I rush to the loo to spit it out and expect to be sick, but this does not happen. I am not in pain, but do not feel comfortable. Since starting the acid suppressant Zantac I have not had any more attacks.

EPISODIC NAUSEA

Query 70-year-old Mrs A.B. from Cardigan writes:

> For the last few years I have had episodes that may last weeks or months where *on waking and sitting up in bed I am overwhelmed by feelings of nausea and the desire to bring up wind*. I have no appetite and have to force myself to eat, but even then can lose a

stone or more in weight. Then quite suddenly for no apparent reason, the symptoms disappear again for weeks and months before a further relapse. I have been investigated from head to toe and been told there is nothing wrong and my symptoms are due to depression. A course of antidepressants exacerbated my symptoms.

Comment There are many possible causes of nausea, including disturbance of the balancing mechanism in the middle ear, which is usually associated with dizziness, or gut problems such as gastritis, gallstones and constipation. When, however, investigation fails to identify an underlying cause, two possible explanations should be considered. The symptoms could be 'functional', that is induced by some impairment of the movement of the stomach and duodenum. Alternatively, they could be due to hypersensitivity of the nerves in the lining of the stomach that generate the sensations of nausea.

(i) *Functional* Several drugs relieve nausea by improving the emptying of the stomach and helping to propel its contents forward.

♦ *Maxolon* 'I too suffer from intermittent nausea. I first experienced it back in the 60s when I lost a good deal of weight. Since then I have had intermittent bouts throughout the years. Extensive tests revealed nothing more than an underactive thyroid. My weight dropped from 10 stone to 8 stone and I lost my appetite completely. Over the last couple of years I have been taking first Maxolon and now Cisapride – three a day. I find this combination helps to control it, but not to cure it. It flares up for a day or two and then settles down, whereas before each bout lasted for weeks or months on end.'

♦ Other drugs that have also been recommended are Domperidone and the powerful anti-nausea drug Ondansetron.

(ii) *Hypersensitivity* If the nerves in the lining of the stomach are 'overtuned', they may misinterpret the presence of normal amounts of acid in the stomach as excessive, inducing in turn the sensation of nausea. Hence acid-suppressant drugs such as Ranitidine should be effective in controlling the nausea.

There are, in addition, several further causes for episodic nausea.

(iii) *Coeliac Disease* Nausea may be a symptom of coeliac disease due to sensitivity to wheat. 'Cutting out all wheat products from my diet has dramatically reduced my nausea. It is hard forsaking bread though!'

(iv) A *'healthy diet'* Current recommendations for a 'healthy' diet include increasing the amount of fibre consumed, which increases the volume of the stool but can also be a cause of nausea.

> My digestion has never been particularly good but it has become steadily worse over the last two years and when I have it in particular I have suffered a lot of nausea. Eventually I saw my doctor, who organized a few tests which were negative. I then asked if he thought my diet could be at fault and told him what a lot of fibre I was eating every day. He told me what a bad irritant too much fibre could be and suggested I should adjust my diet accordingly. It worked like magic. Within two days my symptoms were 85 per cent less and although occasionally I do get a little bit of nausea, I feel so much fitter.'

(v) *Spinal problems* The sensory nerves to the stomach arise from the spinal cord between the shoulder blades, which if compressed may cause nausea that can be relieved by spinal manipulation. Dr A.N. Clapham from Lanark writes:

> When nausea and repetitive burping is associated with back pain this is probably due to problems with the thoracic vertebrae. I had this, right out of the blue, about 25 years ago. In the best traditions of general practice I treated myself for three weeks with all the usual anti-ulcer medications with no effect at all. I then went to see an osteopath who manipulated the relevant joints and I have had no problems since. I have subsequently seen a number of patients with the same problem and I have been able to help many of them in the same way.

Check your Pulse!

There was one further suggestion for unexplained nausea quite distinct from those mentioned above: 'I suffered from episodes of nausea and burping over the last two years. An endoscopy revealed a small hiatus hernia, but an ECG showed that my pulse rate was slowing up and then quickening after the burping.'

Comment This is similar to the mystery cough which similarly synchronized with abnormality of heart rhythm. It is probably mediated through the vagus nerve that travels from the back of the brain down through the chest to the diaphragm. Theoretically, drugs to control the heart rhythm or a pacemaker may be effective.

EPISODIC ABDOMINAL PAIN AND NAUSEA (ABDOMINAL MIGRAINE)

Query 1 Mrs M.L. from Lancashire writing on behalf of her husband writes that for the last four years he has had the most unusual attacks:

> Initially he is *irritable and hungry*. He begins to sniffle as though he has a cold and feels very tired. By the next day he is *queasy, quite often with a temperature, and for several hours vomits a great deal of bile. He is really poorly, but never experiences* any pain. These attacks last for up to 30 hours and after a day to restore his strength, he is fit and well again. We have lost count of the number of fruitless visits to specialists. It would give my husband a great boost if you could find someone with the same syndrome.

Query 2 Mrs B.L. from Sutton Coldfield writes:

> I have some warning as I usually feel unwell for about 24 hours. The actual onset can be very rapid, beginning with *violent nausea*. Within 20 minutes I become totally weak and have to stay perfectly still. My vision goes blurred, I feel terribly nauseous and *cannot tolerate noise or strong light*. I would not have believed it possible to feel so awful. The attack lasts usually about six hours,

during which I am 'totally white faced' and afterwards I am left exhausted with a headache. This has been going on for the last three years and has confounded countless consultants. I feel as though I have reached the end of the line.

Comment There was little doubt that this is abdominal migraine, where vomiting is the main symptom, without the usual headache. Abdominal migraine is well documented in children but there is some doubt that it occurs in adults, which is rather surprising as the first description – back in 1873 – described a man in his 40s:

> The pain began with a deep, ill-defined uneasiness in the epigastrum (stomach) gradually becoming a dull but at first bearable pain. This steadily increased in severity during the next two to three hours until it reached a degree of intensity and then declined. When at its height the pain was intolerable, sickening, and I should say peculiarly visceral in character of the quality produced by a blow in the stomach or testicle and had no griping character whatever. It was always accompanied by chilliness, cold extremities, a slow pulse and a sense of nausea. When the pain began to decline there was generally a feeling of movement in the bowels and perhaps a slight febrile reaction (fever). The paroxysm left very considerable tenderness at the affected region which took a day or two to wear off.

If doctors are still sceptical about the existence of abdominal migraine in adults – despite this well-documented case from over 100 years ago – those who suffer the attacks certainly are not and have little hesitation in saying so.

♦ 'These symptoms will be recognized only too well by many migraine sufferers. They suffer bad temper, hunger (or odd food cravings), tiredness (or hyperactivity) in the build up to an attack. Vomiting, with bile, often comes during attacks. It does sound remarkably like migraine without the headache.'
♦ 'During my 40s I began to suffer from similar symptoms. At first they often started when I was a few days into a holiday, feeling sick, temperature, aches, feeling lousy, irritable, severe headache . . . It really felt as though I was

going down with flu. I would feel completely washed out the next day and then feel reasonably OK. After a number of years and as a result of comparing these symptoms with those of friends, I realized I was suffering from migraine. This had never occurred to me, as I had never had any visual disturbances and I had always thought these were an essential part of migraine attacks.'

♦ 'For about the last 20 years I have suffered from occasional similar attacks – only mine seem worse! It's not just that I have headache and sickness but I am feeling terribly ill: I am incapable of doing or thinking anything and I can barely even bring myself to speak. Even after the first sickness I have to keep rushing to the bathroom although only bile comes up. I can't keep water down. The attack lasts for about ten hours and I have to lie in bed in a darkened room until it passes. Afterwards I feel weak for about another 12 hours but I can then eat and drink little.'

Treatment Treatment is as for the classical migraine attack.

(i) Avoid precipitating factors

♦ *Diet*: Dr D. Bentley from London's Middlesex Hospital reports that in a study of 12 children with abdominal migraine, ten became free or had markedly diminished symptoms after excluding eggs, dairy produce and chocolate – and in some, tea, coffee and citrus fruits – from their diet.

♦ *Driving*: A couple of readers comment that travelling, whether by train or car, can bring on an attack.

(ii) Medication

♦ *Cafergot suppositories*: 'My doctor made a provisional diagnosis of migraine and prescribed Cafergot suppositories, saying that if they worked it would prove the diagnosis. They did work.'

♦ *Aspirin*: Aspirin can abort a migraine headache quite

apart from its analgesic properties. It is interesting to note that it is similarly effective in abdominal migraine. 'I have had recurrent episodes of dyspepsia – loss of appetite, feeling knocked out, etc. These lasted only 24 hours after which I recovered completely. If it started in the evening I had a restless night and often an episode of dry retching first thing in the morning. I tried many things, all to no avail. During one attack I happened to take an aspirin for a toothache or some such thing and my gastric symptoms subsided very rapidly. Thereafter at the first sign I take aspirin, later substituting ibuprofen and the problem was solved.' (It is important to exclude other causes of nausea and vomiting – such as gastritis – which can of course be exacerbated by aspirin).

♦ *Sumatriptan*: This specific anti-migraine drug can abort an acute attack – or if taken as a preventive measure, reduce their frequency.

♦ *Feverfew*: 'Abdominal migraine is more difficult to treat than the usual migraine remedies, but I find Feverfew tablets quite helpful.'

The following two mysteries are probably variants of abdominal migraine.

Query 1 Mrs C.M. from Somerset writes: 'Two to four times a year I get the following symptoms:

Day 1 – sudden onset of extreme tiredness and slight nausea
Day 2 – pain around the lowest right rib increasing over the next three or four days, nausea increases, no vomiting. At worst the soreness and tenderness creeps up the chest slightly to the left of the sternum
Day 6 – begin to feel much better, nausea disappears and pains begin to subside
Day 7–14 – gradually return to full appetite and energy.'

Query 2 'For the last three years I have had the following attacks on and off and although every test has been done, both internally and externally, nobody seems to know what is causing them. The main symptoms are feeling of nausea but no vomiting, shaking as if in shock followed by diarrhoea, complete loss of appetite and weakness and aches in the calf muscles.'

ABDOMINAL PAIN ON MOVEMENT AND LIFTING

Query Mrs C.A., a 53-year-old rent officer from Bournemouth, writes:

> My main problem is the *inability to move around without abdominal pain*. The pain is linked to the muscle down the front right-hand side of my body. *I cannot even pick up a kettle or a plate without discomfort*. I do not drive because I cannot turn the steering wheel and find it difficult to be a passenger in a car because of the vibrations and uneven road surface. I cannot garden or do housework. If I do, and I have tried to over the months, I am invariably in trouble for about 36 hours before it calms down. I am always in discomfort but it is bearable if I keep my body still. I do not get any back pain.

Comment There were two possible suggestions for this most distressing complaint.

Abdominal Hernia

Dr Donald MacLennan, a surgeon at the University of Melbourne, describes a similar case:

> This 27-year-old professional footballer and farmer had a three-year history of right lower abdominal pain. It only occurred when he was playing football or engaged in heavy work on the farm, e.g. lifting bales of hay. Despite intensive ultrasound and heat treatment physiotherapy and steroid injections, the pain persisted and latterly has been taking a few days to fully subside. On examination tenderness could be elicited to deep palpation, but no masses nor defects were found. In view of the worsening abdominal pain and the increasing incapacity an exploratory operation was performed. On retracting the right rectus muscle a hernia sac was encountered large enough to admit a finger. The sac was emptied of contents and excised. Post-operative recovery was uneventful

and the patient was soon back at training and farm work with no recurrence of his symptoms.

Spinal Pain

I have had a similar problem with the same connection to driving and lifting objects of more than a kilogram or so. A tummy pain similar to a stitch would also occur in bed, holding a book and bending to pick up something. It could hardly be classified as disabling, but at worst was irritatingly restrictive and repeatedly peaked from time to time over a period of three years. My doctor diagnosed a trapped nerve and suggested I consult the physiotherapist, who with remarkable insight and prodding skill found the source of the trauma of the nerves. This was surmised to be a dislodged facet joint of the spinal column. Her prescription was forceful flexure exercises of the spine and anti-clockwise torsional flexure. The results were magical within about ten days and remained so after nearly a year, so I am hopeful it may prove permanent.

NOCTURNAL ABDOMINAL DISCOMFORT

Query Mrs R.B. from Stanmore writes:

I am a 60-year-old married woman and have suffered for a number of years from disturbing symptoms which have baffled many specialists. They manifest themselves every night in the form of *extremely strong sensations and discomfort across the stomach area, starting about two hours after going to bed, and they become so stressful that I have to get up and walk about.* They often return again and can sometimes last until the early hours of the morning. I have been prescribed a number of proprietory medicines such as codeine and of course sedatives, and none have been effective. All the usual X-rays and scans have revealed no abnormality. I am desperate to obtain some form of relief. I have suffered from epilepsy for 30 years which has been adequately controlled by Phenytoin. My neurologists do not believe there is any connection.

Comment This most unusual symptom is strongly suggestive of the symptoms of restless legs, which similarly kick in soon after retiring to bed and for which the only solace that can be obtained is rising and moving about. It can be prevented by appropriate medication, which might be considered in this case. Alternatively, a reader described a similar set of symptoms, albeit in the pelvis, which responded to the salt magnesium phosphate.

I am 76 and for the last 16 years have had extreme pain in the pelvic region about one and half to two hours after going to bed. It is only temporarily relieved by getting up and walking about when the whole process was repeated ad nauseum. My doctor was sympathetic, and referred me to a gynaecologist, urologist and a bowel man, who in turn made extensive tests, all to no avail. By chance I came across a book on the use of tissue salts and, to be brief, refined them down to one salt in particular, magnesium phosphate. Use of these salts takes some time to work, particularly in the case of long-standing problems, but after seven weeks treatment I do feel an improvement and am encouraged to persevere. My own diagnosis of the problem was a muscular cramp or spasm – but this was always greeted with glazed eye syndrome!

Two other suggestions both related to problems within the gut.

A twisted appendix

I suffered severe pains in my stomach at night such as I was unable to stay in bed after about two hours. I could only obtain relief by getting up and walking about. After several months of disturbed rest I was referred to a surgeon. I was being treated for diverticulitis at the time and it was thought that one of the pouches had become infected and this in turn had inflamed an ovary. An exploratory operation was performed and the problem was found to be an obstructed hernia of the bowel caused by a very long and twisted appendix. The surgeon told my husband that this condition was so rare he felt as though he had discovered 'a hen's tooth'. I count myself very fortunate to have been operated on by someone who not only recognized the condition but also knew what to do about it.

Impaired blood supply to the gut

A surgeon from Cheshire writes: 'This is a rare syndrome which is in effect due to intermittent claudication (reduced blood flow) of the arteries to the small intestine. My colleague has had this condition for a number of years and was eventually cured by resection of the affected section of the gut. Very few cases have been reported.'

FLATULENCE AFTER SWIMMING

Query 73-year-old former chartered accountant, Mr R.F. from Sussex, writes:

> I endeavour to swim once a week, not always in the same pool. Although I very rarely swallow any of the pool water it is impossible to avoid my face and lips getting wet! *After every swim I suffer with flatulence and a generally upset stomach*, the symptoms usually appearing within 1–2 hours and taking perhaps two days to disappear even when taking medicine.

There were three possible explanations for this unusual mystery syndrome:

♦ *Swallowed air*: Dr Adrian March of the Winchester Swim School writes: I would suggest his problem is that he is swallowing air, not water. Many swimmers who have not mastered a correct breathing technique lack confidence in their ability to take a breath when they want it, consequently they either never exhale properly or they take the largest possible breath and hold it for as long as possible. In either case the consequences are typically as you describe.

Similarly: 'It could well be that in trying to avoid getting lips and face wet he is gulping and swallowing air. He might try the Gruhnberg breathing method (basically breathing in through the mouth then swimming through the water breathing out through the nose).'

♦ *Chlorine sensitivity*: Chlorine could be the answer: 'I cannot drink or wash my hair in heavily chlorinated water as I get awful colic.'

♦ *Type of pool*: I swim in two local pools, one is big and modern, the other smallish, old and somewhat turbulent. I never seem to get any problems after using the "modern" pool, but occasionally have similar symptoms after using the smaller one.'

IRRITABLE BOWEL SYNDROME

Irritable bowel syndrome (IBS) is a dustbin diagnosis for a variety of lower bowel symptoms that at one time were thought to be psychological, as all the usual bowel investigations are normal. These symptoms are now understood to be functional – that is, to do with abnormal functioning of the bowel wall.

The bowel is in a state of constant movement as the muscles in its wall contract and relax, impelling their contents onwards. This wave-like motion is absent in those with irritable bowel syndrome. As a result, they suffer alternately from either constipation – where the bowel is inert – or diarrhoea – where it is overactive, with colicky pains and an excess of wind. No single cause of IBS has been identified, but the severity of the symptoms can be exacerbated by certain foods while stress is certainly a contributory factor.

There are many proprietary preparations available from the chemist for one or other of the several symptoms – laxatives for constipation, anti-diarrhoeal drugs for diarrhoea, charcoal tablets for wind and peppermint-based products for colic. These may alleviate the symptoms, but fail to address whether or not there might be some hidden underlying factor that, were it identified and controlled, would abolish the condition.

Food

♦ *Food sensitivity*: Many different types of food have been incriminated as causing or exacerbating symptoms of IBS. These include high-fibre foods such as bread and cereals; flatus inducing foods such as beans, as well as cabbage, spouts, broccoli, cauliflower and onions; acidic foods including oranges, grapefruits and vinegary salads;

coffee and, surprisingly, lettuce. '*I suffered for years from what the medics thought was IBS until I took myself in hand and started eliminating various foods*, eventually coming to the conclusion that lettuce was the culprit. I had no more trouble until I organized a buffet party and joined in finishing up the delicious sandwiches. Guess what they had in them – lettuce! I took to my bed for a couple of days but have never touched it since and never had a recurrence.'

♦ *Lactose intolerance*: The inability to absorb the sugar lactose in milk and dairy products results in an increased quantity of food residues entering the colon, where they are fermented by colonic bacteria. This results in excess gas production and other symptoms of IBS: 'Between the ages of 18 and 35 I suffered from what was termed irritable bowel. No matter what I tried, I could not alleviate the symptoms. Then the condition vastly improved after a two-week stay at a hotel in Spain. I analysed everything I could think of that might have made a difference while I was away. The only important factor was that I had drunk only sterilized milk, as that was all the hotel provided. I then changed to sterilized milk at home and the vast improvement continued. I now feel sad I was debilitated for such a long period of my life.'

♦ *Coeliac disease (wheat sensitivity)*: The gluten component of wheat can damage the lining of the small bowel producing IBS-type symptoms. 'For many years I endured the symptoms of irritable bowel, all the while believing that bread was such a fundamental in a staple diet it must be good for everyone. However, I read by chance a recipe which suggested ground rice as a thickener for those who wanted to avoid gluten and, out of curiosity, I stopped my intake of all foods derived from cereals. The effect on my bowel function was immediate and totally beneficial. I did on one occasion return to eating bread and just as immediately my bowel problem recurred.'

♦ *Soya flour*: Alternatively, some people may be sensitive to the soya flour present in bread: 'My wife had irritable bowel syndrome, discomfort, wind and looseness. She had all the investigations and was given the all-clear. For some reason she noticed our usual wholemeal bread had soya flour in it. If you look you will find that nearly all cereal (mass-produced bakery) products have soya in. It is difficult to find any without. My wife succeeded in discovering a bread with no soya and has had no problem since except when, by accident, she ate some biscuits containing it and it recurred. I would suggest that as a first step to cutting out cereals people cut out those with soya. After all it is a bean and all little boys know what beans means!'

Fluoride and Aluminium

Several readers identified a sensitivity to fluoride or aluminium cooking pots as a factor in their symptoms:

♦ 'I recently read that there are more than 8 million sufferers of irritable bowel in the UK. Purely by accident, a few months ago, I discovered a link between fluoride and IBS. I found that when I switched to a non-fluoride toothpaste and used bottled water, my cramps, bloating, diarrhoea and exhaustion disappeared. If I drink tap water my symptoms return within 24 hours.'

♦ 'My husband used to have IBS. I bought a Kenwood water filter machine, since when he has had minimal trouble although if he eats chocolate he does suffer. His severe and chronic IBS was cured within 4–5 weeks by throwing away all aluminium cooking utensils and using stainless steel instead. I was recommended to do this by my family doctor.'

Bile Acid Sensitivity

The bile acids produced by the gall bladder can, for some people, have a purgative effect, causing particularly severe diarrhoea. This is more likely to occur in those who have had their gall bladder removed or other abdominal operations, and can be dramatically cured by a drug, Questran, which mops them up.

After repeated bursts of severe diarrhoea I consulted my family doctor, who diagnosed IBS and prescribed anti-diarrhoea medication. The bouts continued for no apparent reason and I was referred to a consultant, who advised that everything in my gut was in order and therefore IBS was the likely cause. The diarrhoea continued. It was severe, painful and unpredictable. I dared not arrange social events and holidays. I read books and leaflets on IBS and tried high fibre, low fibre, exclusion diets and complementary medicine – all to no avail. After a further year and one and a half stones lighter, I was referred to a second consultant. He listened to my story and noticed in particular I had had my gall bladder removed two years earlier. He suggested that I may be sensitive to bile acid and prescribed Questran twice a day. The result was instant relief. My diarrhoea has ceased and I have regained my lost weight and social life.

APRIL BOWEL

Query Mr C.C. from Hertfordshire writes:

I call my condition 'April bowel' and no one has been able to find a cure. *When the weather is unsettled and especially when rain is threatening, my stomach and bowel are also unsettled although not nauseous.* I feel slightly better when I eat. My condition is accompanied by lethargy and feeling dozy and tired and everything takes longer because I have to think with great care what I am doing. As soon as it becomes sunny and warm all these symptoms vanish as if they had never been. As my 'April bowel' would seem to be a function of our English weather I have been considering that it might be better to move to Spain for a permanent remedy.

Comment Several further examples of weather-related bowel and other afflictions were volunteered:

♦ 'I have found I am affected very much by any rapid drop in barometic pressure and particularly by the approach of rain or snow. The atmospheric symptoms usually take the form of a tightness or inflammation of muscles within the rib cage and around the heart, causing *flatulence and shallow breathing, poor concentration and an extreme state of agitation and inability to relax*, so sleep is out of the question. The onset of rain can mostly bring almost immediate relief, though in the interim I do have to resort to ibuprofen for some solace. In winter the advent of snow can be forecast, even when it is far distant, by a full, boring ache in my chest muscles through to my back. Strangely enough, the rest of the time I enjoy a reasonably healthy life.'

♦ 'I have suffered from catarrh and sinus problems since I was young. These days the sinus condition mostly seems to be brought on by the change of wind direction, i.e. from the north-west or sometimes from the north-east. When this happens my sinuses are completely blocked; when the warmer winds return I can breathe more freely.'

♦ 'I have had a rheumatic condition for many years. My husband made the observation I am worse when the wind is in the north-east for some inexplicable reason! By chance I learnt that if I went to the west country on holiday I was worse and to the east I was much better, hence our move from Dorset to Canterbury when we retired four years ago and where I have been considerably better. Tangible proof of the effect of weather came last month when I visited my physiotherapist for my routine 'service'. The weather had been wet for some time and when she came to manipulate my hip she could not move it at all. She did not have the time to spend on it at that appointment and I had to go back in a week by which time the weather had cleared and my leg nearly came off in her hand! In damp weather my joints swell and I feel decidedly sinusy. There is a general feeling of malaise – indeed I have sometimes taken my temperature as I feel so fluy.'

The reasons for these weather-related symptoms are certainly likely to be complex, but the following suggestions were made.

Howard Tarey of Malvern reports that a few hours before the weather changes from clear to overcast with rain, he notices a loss of appetite, slight sinus pain, dizziness and difficulty in concentrating. As soon as the rain passes, so do the symptoms. Mr Tarey is a physicist and in the spirit of scientific enquiry has examined the possibilities.

It is clearly atmospheric. Some causes, however, can be excluded. Barometic pressure would seem to be implicated but the timing is not right; symptoms occur before a fall in pressure and disappear before it rises again. Neither do temperature or humidity seem to be involved. Ionization is a possibility but a commercial ionizer does not help. I suspect an agent is released from damp soil, plants or surfaces by rain which is then blown in the direction the rain is heading.

Dr Diana Samways from Haslemere suggests a similar explanation:

I had a combination of mood swings, arthritis of large joints, bowel problems and severe loss of energy with flu-like symptoms which occurred seasonally, worse in March and August, and were undoubtedly triggered by wet weather and damp. This was often set off by a thunderstorm or period of stormy wind and I too relate it to atmospheric pressure changes. I came to the conclusion my ill health was due to allergy to inhaling mould spores prior to thunderstorms and other low-pressure phenomena, and damp weather. These are greatly increased in April when lawn mowing starts. The first cut liberates a massive increase in mould spores into the air which we then breathe in.

RECTAL PAIN

Query Mr T.J., a 60-year-old retired company director from Kent, writes:

For the last nine years I have suffered from perianal (around the anus) pain. It started quite suddenly and was first thought to be an anal fissure. When that was ruled out I ended up seeing virtually every type of consultant from orthopaedic to neurologist by way of general surgeons and urologists and have had all sorts of investigations from X-rays to MRI scans. None of these has shown any abnormalities. The pain is debilitating and varies in intensity from mild discomfort to putting me in bed with an icepack for a day or two. My mobility is impaired as walking makes it worse and the thought of riding a bicycle or running for a bus is out of the question. I have been prescribed Amitriptyline as a long-term pain suppressor, but that brings its own problems. Consequently the quality of life is degraded and looks like continuing that way. The only diagnosis guessed at is that there is something wrong with the coccyx and the treatment an operation to remove it. I am naturally reluctant to embark on such a major step.

Comment There are several types of rectal pain, each of which has quite specific symptoms and appropriate treatment.

Stabbing pains – proctalgia fugax (fleeting pain in the rectum)

This is much the commonest type of rectal pain, which affects one in ten of the adult population and is believed to be due to a spasm of the muscles of the anal sphincter. It often wakes the sufferer at night.

♦ 'My attacks usually happen in the middle of the night such as 3.00 a.m. I would be wakened by a slight pain and will get to know what will follow and get myself out of bed. The pain would increase steadily through five minutes or so, stay that way for another five or ten and then subside slowly. At its height it was awful. All I could do was walk up and down the hall and round and round the sitting room trying not to scream.'

♦ 'The pain comes on at any old time – when typing, or walking, or doing household chores – even sleeping. It begins with one just a little warning – quite mild – the way I try to explain it is as if one hears a train in the very far distance and then it steadily comes towards the 'station', ever increasing in noise (pain) and roaring through.

The peak of the pain lasts for me between 15 and 30 minutes and then it very gradually eases. It is quite a draining experience.'

♦ 'Both my wife and myself and my ten-year-old daughter suffer from what I call anal neuralgia, which occasionally wakens us in the night but more usually comes on after defecation. It starts as a dull ache, rapidly increasing to an almost intolerable pain in the rectum.'

Treatment

(i) *Heat and cold*: Very hot baths or a hot water bottle can effectively abort an attack as indeed does ice.

• 'Heat seems to be the only remedy, but it is uncomfortable and inconvenient to have to rise in the night to have to prepare hot water.'

• 'My problem has been around for about six years and I find that sitting over the toilet with ice wrapped in an old handkerchief is very helpful.'

• 'When we got a refrigerator I would put a lump of ice into the rectum. I went to see the doctor, who suggested I had some sex complex after years of being on my own.'

• 'I have found a small self-administered enema of very cold water stops the pain sooner than anything, especially if it is followed by absolute stillness in the recumbent position.'

(ii) *Dilating the anus*:

• 'I have suffered from this intense pain for years. My doctor told me it was due to anal spasms and prescribed an anal dilator. It's a sort of small glass carrot shaped device which I insert with the help of KY jelly. It always works and as the pain fades I fall into a very deep sleep.'

• 'I was advised to perform a digital rectal examination on myself. It relieves the pain most effectively. The idea was that it was due to spasm in the region of the sphincter and stretching the muscle alleviated the spasm.'

(iii) *Bearing down*:

• 'I find that when this painful spasm occurs, bearing down as if passing a motion brings total relief in seconds.'

(iv) *Alcohol*:

• 'Both myself and my wife suffer from acute pains of the rectum that occur for no apparent reason but can be cured almost instantly by drinking a small glass of dry sherry.'

• 'What works for me now is half a glass of Guinness drunk very quickly. The wind comes up almost immediately. I can then go back to bed pain free.'

• 'My family doctor suggested brandy and that really did help. It's always a little embarrassing if the pain starts in the office. Even if one took the flask to the ladies and returning smelling of brandy!'

(v) *Medication*:

• *Preventative painkillers*: 'I found some relief with a combination of paracetemol and codeine by taking them late at night. I also found they helped me to sleep.'

• *GTN*: 'My family doctor suggested glycerine trinitrate. These are horrible tablets which can give a terrible headache. They work wonders.'

• *Salbutamol*: Dr J.E. Wright from Australia writes: 'The stimulus for trying Salbutamol inhalation arose during discussion with the mother of a young boy who had typical bouts of proctalgia nightly for four or five nights recurring every six months or so. The pain was described as muscle spasm and the mother asked if it was like labour pain. Because of the effects of Salbutamol in labour it was decided to try Salbutamol inhaler during the boy's next attack. He obtained relief almost instantly. The pain recurred an hour and a half later, but again relief followed the inhalation of Salbutamol. As I have had proctalgia fugax for many years I tried the same treatment. Relief was obtained within a few minutes with a few good puffs of Salbutamol and there was no recurrence.'

Hereditary Rectal Pain

There is a hereditary form of rectal pain – similar to proctalgia fugax – that runs in families which, like the facial pain of trigeminal neuralgia, is elicited by stimulation of a trigger point in the rectum, resulting in a lancinating pain. Dr Richard Duggan from Wisconsin writes:

This pain accompanies a bowel movement or may follow a fall on the buttocks on probing in the anal region. Those affected assess this as the worst pain they have ever known. It *begins near the anus, shoots down one of the legs and reaches the feet in the more intense reactions.* The duration is less than a minute and following it the person is usually fatigued. In the immediate aftermath, the flesh reddens on the buttocks and genitals. The flushing spreads rapidly down the frontal surface of one or both legs and begins to encircle the leg.

It has been described as follows:

It is a terrible pain that affects the bottom and legs when going to the toilet. It does not always occur. It is very hard to explain but starts like an itch which then turns to a terrible burning sensation which gets worse and worse, spreading to the whole of the lower part of the body, travelling down the back of the legs to the heel of the foot, turning the skin bright red which takes about an hour to get back to normal. It is really a terrible pain which gives you a continual fear all your life.

Treatment The treatment, as with trigeminal neuralgia, is the anti-epileptic drug Tegretol.

Foreign Bodies in the Rectum

♦ 'I suffered from occasional anal pain over a number of years. It was always acute and came on during the night. Although only occasional, I tried to discover the reason for it and came to the conclusion this always happened after eating peanuts. Not cashews which are a softer nut. Cut out the hard, brittle, jagged edge peanuts, no anal pain.'

♦ Dr D.H. Davies of Cardiff's Royal Infirmary reports the following case: 'A 31-year-old male presented to the casualty with a nine-hour history of severe rectal pain. He was obviously in distress, unable to sit without experiencing the excruciating rectal pain. On examination he was found to have a hard sharp object lodged horizontally just above the anal margin. He was sedated and a 4cm long bone fragment was removed. On further questioning he recalled eating chicken 48 hours prior to the onset of the pain.'

Anal Pain with Numbness

Those whose anal pain is associated with numbness and is worse on sitting and lying and relieved by standing may have compression of the pudendal nerve. Dr John Bascom from Oregon writes: 'Eight patients reported *anal pain on sitting and, strikingly an identical intense pain on lying down.* Standing always abolished or diminished the pain. All patients experienced temporary pain relief with a nerve block and four patients received longer relief by surgical decompression.'

Tender Coccyx (Coccydynia)

Dr Linda Frazier from Duke University Medical Centre writes:

> Four years ago a 39-year-old woman fell, *hitting her coccyx* on the edge of a landscaping beam. The severe pain subsided after several weeks, but *intermittent pain exacerbated by sitting or prolonged standing remained.* She had a habit of sitting with her feet propped up on a stool. There was marked tenderness on palpation of the coccyx. X-rays showed no fracture. A diagnosis of coccydynia was made. She was advised to sit on a donut pillow and use a shorter chair. During two years of follow-up the symptoms waxed and waned.

Rectal 'Dull Ache' (the Levator Syndrome)

Dr Stewart Grant of New Jersey writes: 'The levator syndrome consists of *pain, pressure or discomfort in the region of the rectum, sacrum and coccyx that are often increased by sitting.*'

Most patients complain of vague, indefinite rectal discomfort or pain which is described as being high in the rectum. A feeling of rectal pressure may accompany the pain or may be present alone. Some may complain of feeling a 'ball' or other intrarectal object. In addition some may experience severe pain awakening them from sleep, as occurs in proctalgia fugax. The diagnosis is made by a demonstration of tenderness and muscle spasm affecting the levator muscles. Most patients obtain relief with treatment with massage, diathermy or baths and muscle relaxants.

10
Smells

Body odours have only a minor influence on human social activity – in marked contrast to the rest of the animal world – except in the most general sense where different types of diet influence smell and so encourage mating within one social and racial group. It has always been a matter of curiosity to Europeans and Americans that the Chinese claim Westerners have a distinct unpleasant smell of sour milk. Ellis Douek, formerly of Guy's Hospital and great odour expert, reports how a group of Chinese women returning home from the United States to find a husband insisted as soon as they boarded ship on eating only Chinese food. They explained it would take several days before they lost their 'Western' smell.

Human odours have a useful biological function only in infancy – to compensate for the lack of development of the other senses. They help babies find their source of food while encouraging mothers to love their babies. Dr Heili Varendi from Tartu University in Estonia reported an ingenious experiment in *The Lancet* where 30 mothers, immediately after delivery were asked to wash one breast thoroughly with an odourless liquid while leaving the other untouched. Their newborn babies were then placed faced down between the breasts. Virtually all rooted to the unwashed side. 'Naturally occurring maternal odours from the breast may have a role in guiding infants to the nipple, and thereby contributing to early suckling and attachment,' Dr Varendi concluded.

Just as maternal smells help an infant find the nipple, so the infant's smell binds the mother to the baby. This is believed to be the explanation for the quite characteristic smell exuded by babies in the first six months – often described as being like 'crumpets' or 'vanilla' – which encourages mothers to kiss them often and enthusiastically.

By contrast, evil odours can be a source of much distress and come in several forms – strong cheese odour, acidy odour, rotten food odour, fetal odour, strong sweat odour, fish smell, halitosis and vaginal malodour. This section starts with total body malodour and then goes on to consider its origins from other specific sites.

BODY MALODOUR

At one time, distinctive body odours provided essential clues to the cause of infectious illness. Thus surgeons working on British soldiers fighting for the empire in the nineteenth century suspected yellow fever if the patient exuded the smell of a butcher's shop. If the armpits of someone with a rash of fever exuded the aroma of freshly baked bread, doctors would confidently diagnose a case of typhoid fever. When diphtheria was endemic, a discriminating physician could pick out a case from a queue of 60 children because of the characteristic sweetish odour. In the field hospitals of the First World War, surgeons were alert to the pervasive stench of rotten apples – indicating gangrene. If a wound gave off a sweet whiff of grapes, it had been infected with the bacterium pseudomina.

These exotic diseases are rarely seen nowadays and the physician's olfactory diagnostic skills are limited to a handful of rare diseases of childhood due to inborn errors of metabolism. These include the mousey smell of phenylketonuria, the sweet smell of maple syrup urine disease; the offensive odour of sweaty feet syndrome; the dead fish smell of fish odour syndrome; the rancid butter smell of rancid butter syndrome; and the yeast-like smell of oast house urine disease. We consider here four further mystery body odours.

Kipper Smell

Query Mr R.C. from Sherborne writes:

> Over the past few months I have suffered from a problem that causes me no small embarrassment. Often after typing letters or concentrating on money problems, *I become aware on rising from my seat of a distinct odour of kippers*. I have on numerous occasions examined my urine and also weep stains in my pants, but have failed to locate any source of this odour. The GP has been unable to suggest any cause.

Comment There seems little doubt that the source of the kipper smell is a type of light fitting or other electrical appliance which when heated gives off this unpleasant odour.

♦ 'I came across this problem 40 years ago in the bathroom of a new house I had recently moved into. The stench was overwhelming and I quickly decided there was a leak from the toilet seeping under the floor covering and quietly fermenting. How wrong I was, but I had dismantled the toilet and ruined the floor covering before I tracked down the source of the odour by literally by following my nose. It came from the lamp holder of the light fitting, which was subject to great heat from the bulb. It seems that many types of lampholder are made from plastic containing urea which, under high temperatures, gives off this obnoxious odour.'

♦ 'Last week when a friend visited I apologized for the smell of fish in my kitchen while the dishwasher was operating and blamed a dodgy packet of new dishwasher detergent tablets. He went straight to attempt to unplug the machine but cried out because of the heat which almost burnt his fingers. He had experienced a similar smell/stink with a washing machine. When the plug had cooled and been dismantled the wires were still attached. The plastic coating was melting and emitting an obnoxious smell of fish. The cable was shortened, a new plug fitted and the smell has gone.'

There were, in addition three further suggestions:

♦ *Fish odour syndrome*: Fish odour syndrome is caused by the inability to break down a chemical, trimethylamine – a biproduct of the protein that gives fish its fishy smell – in the gut. Damaris Christensen explains: 'People with this disorder can release trimethylamine through sweat, breath and urine. A few have a strong odour all the time but most others experience this severe smell that fluctuates over time.' There is no cure for fish odour syndrome, but a special diet can alleviate the worst of the odour problems. This involves a low-protein regime restricting the amino acid choline, a building block of protein naturally found in high concentrations in fish, eggs, beans and organ meats. Some people also report that limiting lecithin, a common food additive also naturally found in eggs, soya beans and corn, also helps reduce the odour. Finally, as bacteria in the gut produce most of the trimethylamine in the body, some people find that low doses of antibiotics, which kill off these bacteria, temporarily suppress the odour.

♦ *Smelly button syndrome*: 'I believe the cause of the kipper smell is smelly tummy button. It is necessary to clean it out well and dry well inside. I have the same problem when wearing a tight belt or sitting down with a tight waist band.'

♦ *Wrist watch syndrome*: 'My secretary was a forthright lady and assured me, when she put her head round the door, that I did not have BO and was not filling with office with a malodour. I sat at my desk with my hand on my chin and heard her in disbelief. Then the penny dropped. The underside of my wrist watch where the strap adjoins collects a jam of sweat and dead skin which effluves when moist and warm.'

Foul Nasal Odour

Dr Irvine Golding of the Pittsburg School of Medicine describes this unusual but eminently treatable 'unbearably foul odour' in an 18-month-old child.

For approximately four weeks he had been emanating an unbearably foul odour from his entire body. No part of his being appeared to be free of the fetid odour. The stench was so inescapable and uniquely obnoxious the mother was developing hostile feelings towards her offspring. Beside the ever-presence of the child's odour, anyone who touched his skin noticed that the body part which was in contact with the boy smelt the same. Bathing the child brought relief only for about 15 minutes. When his clothes were removed they would have the same odour. There was no other evidence of illness and the child maintained a usually good humour and even disposition. On examination there was a definite mass visualized in the nose. A soaked piece of blanket was easily removed with a bayonet forcep. This foreign body had the same odour as that which was coming from the child. An hour later the mother called and reported the odour was indeed gone.

Smelly Scalp

Query A 43-year-old woman from South Wirral writes:

Since my first baby 17 years ago, I have suffered from what I describe as 'smelly scalp' syndrome. I wash my hair every day, sometimes twice, but *after only a few hours my scalp smells and feels as though it has not been washed for days*. It has got a horrible greasy smell and my scalp feels greasy. I get very embarrassed as I am very aware of it and hate getting too near to people. I have had two more children since then and the problem has been with me all the time, getting worse when my period is due. The only respite I have had is when I had keyhole surgery for my gall bladder and my scalp stayed sweet smelling all day for about two weeks.

Comment There were three treatment suggestions for this unusual syndrome:

(i) *Anti-dandruff shampoo*: 'Normally my hair needs a weekly wash as it never gets greasy, but some years ago when I purchased a strong dandruff shampoo I only had to use it three times and by then my hair was lank and greasy after a day. It took six months to get back to normal. The scalp reacts to the strong shampoo by secreting even greater volumes of sebum.'

(ii) *Dairy products*: 'Some years ago my husband noticed my scalp had an unpleasant odour, although I was washing my hair daily. He also complained I had halitosis and my skin was putrid. For many years I had suffered from painful joints and was receiving physiotherapy, when it was suggested that the joint pains might be due to an allergy to dairy products. I now drink goats milk and try not to eat so much butter or cheese. I no longer "smell" and my joint pains and stiffness have greatly improved. I am sure if I could manage to give up eating butter and cheese altogether I would feel even better.'

(iii) *Hormones*: 'I have suffered from smelly scalp most of my life. It disappeared overnight as soon as I started to take HRT. Amazing and brilliant. I no longer have to wash my hair daily but can let it go for several days and it now looks (and smells!) good.'

Drugs

Several drugs can cause unusual body odours, including the anti-acne medication benzoyl peroxide, as described by Dr Peter Molberg from Oregon:

A 15-year-old girl was brought to the surgery by her mother for evaluation of a *'peculiar' odour that persisted in her clothes even with washing*. Bedclothes and bedsheets had to be discarded periodically. The patient was using 10 per cent benzoyl peroxide for acne. She was advised to stop using the medication, and a month later her mother happily reported the odour problem was solved. She was asked to resume her acne treatment, and the odour returned within three days. Again, stopping the preparation stopped the odour. Attempts to extract the metabolic product causing the odour was unsuccessful.

HALITOSIS

Query Mr C. from Sussex writes:

My partner and I are both middle aged and she has terrible bad breath. *Since we met some years ago she brushes her teeth after*

every meal – but an hour later her breath smells terrible. Her teeth
are sound but badly discoloured. She goes to a good dentist who
advised her to clean with dental sticks between the teeth, which
she does. I wonder if the smell emanates from the stomach.
Whatever the cause – is there anything that can be done?'

Comment Halitosis is a social killer, even more so nowadays
when standards of personal hygiene are so much higher thanks
to better dental care and the presence of a bath in every home.
The standard line on halitosis is that it is due to poor dental
hygiene, with the implication that it is the sufferer's fault for
neglecting to brush their teeth to get rid of the detritus that
accumulates around the molars. But this is certainly not the
whole story; those who are self-conscious about their bad
breath are probably more assiduous teeth brushers than anyone else, but are still unable to eradicate their antisocial odour.
Nonetheless, most cases of bad breath are due to the presence
of bacteria and their evil-smelling products – even though it
can often be difficult to locate precisely where they are hanging
out. The following possibilities should be considered.

Dental Restoration

Mr W.I. Shear, a dental surgeon in London, reports the following case:

> A 67-year-old male patient attended about two years ago com-
> plaining his wife had detected a very unpleasant mouth odour. It
> was so bad it was most embarrassing. The patient was in excellent
> health. He was told to brush his tongue and palate and put on
> chlorhexidine mouth rinses, but this only controlled the odour for
> a few hours at a time. He recently reattended with the cusp of the
> upper first premolar – which had an amalgam restoration – that
> had fractured off. Since then the mouth odour had completely
> disappeared. I suspect the odour was caused by bacteria within the
> tooth fracture and colonizing under the restoration. If this is so,
> then cracked teeth should be suspected in cases where normal
> measures and investigations (for the control of halitosis) produce
> no results.

Nasal Foreign Body

As in the case outlined above, an intranasal foreign body can also cause bad breath alone. A lady from Stockton writes:

> My three-year-old granddaughter had suffered from *bad breath for almost a year*. She then developed nose bleeds, which the doctor attributed to polyps in her nose. He said if it continued he would need to refer her to hospital for investigation. Subsequently I saw an article discussing foreign bodies as the cause of bad breath. I mentioned to my daughter-in-law that my granddaughter could have pushed something up her nostril. She was referred to the casualty department of the local hospital where a piece of folded shoebox cardboard was removed from the left nostril. The smell has now disappeared and we are all greatly relieved.

Gut Infection

When there is no obvious source of infection in the mouth or upper airways, alternative possibilities must be considered. The most obvious is that the odour might be coming from the gut – though on theoretical grounds this is unlikely as the intense acidity of the stomach destroys 99.9 per cent of bacteria within a few seconds. The exception is a type known as helicobacter, implicated in peptic ulcers, which is ingeniously adapted to survive in this most acidic of environments. There have been several reports that following a course of antibiotics to eliminate these bacteria, patients find their breath smells sweeter.

Drugs

Commonly prescribed drugs can, for reasons unknown, be a cause of bad breath. An American physician reports: 'Several of my patients taking Isosorbide Dinitrate (for the treatment of angina) complained of halitosis which appeared with the onset of therapy, was reversible when therapy was discontinued and recurred when it was resumed.'

Malignancy

Very importantly, halitosis that develops for the first time in those who are 60 or over can be a potentially sinister early sign of malignancy in the mouth or sinuses, and requires thorough investigation to identify its cause.

OFFENSIVE FLATUS

Query 70-year-old Mr S.R. from Southampton writes:

> I do not suffer from indigestion, any other stomach discomfort or trapped wind, but find that *foul smelling flatulence has become an increasing problem.* I have tried wheat-free diets, giving up dairy products, drinking wine, alo vera juice, natural yoghurt. My family doctor has prescribed various peppermint-based tablets and I have tried other products which might help. All to no effect. I obviously avoid things like baked beans or anything which is high fibre. All we can do at the moment is to employ various pleasant smells in the room to counteract the problem.

Comment Flatus is produced by the fermentation by bacteria of undigested food residues in the colon. This offensive flatus usually reflects the composition of the bacteria in the gut. Theoretically it might be influenced by antibiotic therapy and indeed treatment with antibiotics such as Tetracycline, Neomycin and Metronidazole have been reported to have a favourable effect. It is also helpful to know that when visiting friends and relations, lighting a match after a visit to the toilet will eliminate any sulphurous smells left behind. Solicitous hosts will leave a box of matches in the 'little room' for this purpose – though Swan are apparently more effective than safety matches.

VAGINAL MALODOUR

The common cause of vaginal malodour is bacterial vaginosis – a bacterial infection of the vagina – with organisms such as bacteroides. Dr Katherine Forrest, writing in *The Lancet* observes:

Bacterial vaginosis is marked by a thin vaginal discharge and genital malodour. There is hardly any or no inflammation. *The odour usually described as fishy or musty, can be elicited from freshly smeared secretions.* The disease is sexually transmitted, as male partners of women with bacterial vaginosis have greater numbers of bacterial species in urethral specimens. I found that when a woman has recurrent bacterial vaginosis it helps to treat her with oral or vaginal medication and to prescribe oral medication for her male partner.

Dr Morray Zimmerman from California describes the following unusual syndrome of an unpleasant vaginal odour in a 33-year-old woman, induced by sexual arousal: 'She complains of an *extremely unpleasant vaginal odour* that developed subsequent to a hysterectomy two years ago. The odour appears only when she is sexually aroused and seems to be severe enough to affect the happiness of her marriage.'

Dr George Preti of the University of Pennsylvania comments:

The odour of human vaginal secretions has been found to vary in intensity and pleasantness throughout the menstrual cycle. In addition, the odour of these secretions is generally rated as unpleasant by human observers. Many vaginal contraceptive creams have a pleasant smell and, if used prior to coitus, may serve to mask the offensive odour. Alternatively, since production of many odourless compounds is dependent on bacteria, an antibiotic cream may be helpful.

MISCELLANEOUS ODOUR PROBLEMS

Four further distinctive odours have also been described – for which however, no explanations were forthcoming.

Dusty Scent

'About a year ago I began to notice a smell rather similar to the rather dusty scent of an old paperback book. Since I was often reading when the smell appeared, the book or newspaper seemed a likely source, until I noticed that my urine had the same smell and although I have not noticed it on my breath, every other bodily emanation has the same odour. On hot days it has been quite pronounced and it was obvious the sweat glands were playing the same tune. If anyone else has noticed it there has been no comment and everything and everyone smells to me as they always have.'

Yeasty Smell

'Even shortly after a bath, and especially in the morning, I am aware of a yeasty smell on my skin. Others say they do not notice this, but to me this is very apparent.'

Spice

'For the last three months I have been beset with a pungent smell which is clearly coming from me somewhere. It smells like spice and comes in strong waves, a number of times a day when it is either warm indoors or when I get warm doing gardening outside.'

Sweet Smell

Since my husband's death from a stroke I have had a sickly scented smell in my nostrils. I waken during the night with it and my urine, which is perfectly normal, has the same scented smell. I do not have diabetes. My smell is perfectly normal in other respects except when chopping onions – I no longer smell them, whereas before I used to have tears rolling down my face.

11
The Bladder

Common bladder ailments – the pain and increased frequency of cystitis, impeded urinary flow due to an enlarged prostate and so on – are straightforward enough and the treatment for most are quite logical. But with the mystery syndromes described here, the cause can be elusive and with a couple mimicking other well-recognized conditions, it can take a lot of time before things are sorted out.

BASHFUL BLADDER

There is something uniquely embarrassing about going into a crowded public lavatory, waiting for an empty urinal, getting ready to pass urine and then finding nothing happens. Those in close proximity naturally suspect one of being a sexual exhibitionist, so this further heightens the embarrassment and still nothing happens. This is bashful bladder syndrome or, in medical terminology, paruresis. It may seem trivial enough, even blackly humorous, but for those afflicted it is no joke at all – afraid of being ridiculed by others they seek lavatories in out of the way places in the hope they will be allowed to urinate in peace.

Query Mr A.B. from Hertfordshire writes:

> I suffer the complaint to a mild degree, but have acquaintances who admit to a considerable problem in this respect. The great

fear for the sufferer is the open trough urinal and its total lack of privacy. It is unfortunate that this type of urinal is so common and with it the unedifying sight of men shoulder to shoulder splashing, dripping and shaking their penises with the resultant pools of urine soaking into the soles.

Comment Dr Julie Hatterer, psychiatrist at Columbia University, describes two further cases:

♦ 'Mr A., a 38-year-old divorced man, presented with a 30-year history of paruresis. *He was unable to use a public urinal if others were present*, or if others were waiting for his turn to use the restroom. He avoided crowded facilities and limited his fluid intake when going out.'

♦ 'Mr C., a 40-year-old single man, had a 36-year history of being unable to urinate in public facilities and in recent years had developed almost complete phobic avoidance, forcing him to work from home.'

The cause of paruresis is not known, which has not discouraged doctors from putting forward their fanciful theories. It has been suggested that apprehension about penis size – whether too long or too short – may be a factor, but in a survey only three out of a sample of 150 men provided this as a possible explanation. Alternatively, Dr Alan Mayers of the Boston Medical Center, noting the behaviour of those mammalian species in which the male urinates to mark off his territory with his scent, comments: 'Might it be that modern homosapiens who attempt to pass urine in the presence of another male are inhibited by the unconscious message "if I do so I am asserting my claim to this territory – am I ready to challenge others to fight over it?" '

The more sensible view is that this is a peculiar variant of social phobia, an exaggeration of the normal reaction of shyness when even the most straightforward of encounters with strangers is thwarted by a lack of self-confidence. While for obvious reasons, paruresis is widely perceived as being primarily a male complaint, women too may similarly be self-conscious – though here the inhibition to passing urine is acoustic rather than visual: although out of sight of the person in the next cubicle, a woman may feel apprehensive that the tinkle of her urine into the bowl will be overheard.

This proved a serious problem for one woman, who had to contribute a urine specimen as part of a drug screening programme at her place of work. She was unable to perform in the room where testing was taking place and by way of encouragement was told to drink water. Despite knocking back almost three litres in an hour, she was still unable to perform and so was sent home, where she became confused, her speech slurred and gait unsteady. On admission to hospital she was found to be suffering from acute water intoxication, with swelling of the brain. Luckily she recovered without complication.

Treatment Treatment is not very satisfactory, as drugs such as the beta blockers commonly used in the treatment of social phobia do not seem to be of much value. However, behaviour modification, and in particular the technique of cognitive therapy, has its advocates. Other suggestions include:

(i) *Visualization*: A reader recalls watching an American police drama on television where a number of officers had been asked to provide urine samples for random drugs tests. 'A young detective was having difficulty delivering the goods. "Shy bladder, huh?" said his older colleague standing next to him. "I imagine a bowling ball rolling down the alley – works every time for me." And it has done ever since for me.'

(ii) *Cold water*: 'My father, a doctor, told me to run my wrist under a cold tap.'

(iii) *Music*: 'We were fortunate on a visit to Tokyo to have a friend working out there. She took us out and about, including a visit to a big hotel on Tokyo Bay. My wife was intrigued by an unmarked button in the ladies loo. Our friend explained it was a "modesty button", when pressed soft music played to hide the noise of the tinkle!'

'ELECTRIC SHOCK' ON URINATION

Query 1 80-year-old Mrs S.B. from Suffolk writes: 'I suffer from bouts of cystitis from time to time and although the discomfort of constantly needing to spend a penny is rather trying, the puzzling and rather painful sensation is that of *acute pricking in my hands as I pass urine*. This pricking is pretty powerful, almost like a *mild electric current* passing through my hand.

Query 2 Mrs M.B. from Dorset writes: 'I experience a *sharp electric shock type pain when passing urine*. It travels rapidly from the fingertips to the elbow on my right hand. After several days it ceases for several months and then recurs with no warning. I had the impression that my family doctor didn't really believe me when I once mentioned it.'

Query 3 'The pain floods up my body from the bladder and down my arms, finishing up in the palms of my hands with a tingling sensation. I have mentioned this to doctors, nurses and friends and no one knows what I am talking about.'

Comment This electric shock sensation in the hands is most commonly associated with the bladder infection known as cystitis. Some readers also say it occurs when they have to 'hold on' before being able to go to the toilet. It is very difficult to explain for the obvious reason that there are no nerves linking the bladder with the hands. It could, however, be a variant of the 'referred pain' as described in the Introduction and in Chapter 18, A Clutch of Curiosities.

There were a couple of suggestions that it might be related to pressure on the nerves in the spine, but this was disputed.

♦ 'I went to my family doctor, who professed puzzlement but thought it must be a problem with my neck and suggested I might consider visiting an osteopath. With some trepidation I made a booking, but quickly received treatment to my neck with almost immediate relief. I was shown how to keep it upright with the chin held in –

though it is difficult to use the average urinal with any great accuracy from this position. While not yet entirely cured, I am now aware of the cause and can control what I would at times describe as this excruciating pain.'

♦ 'Some time ago I became aware of this weird feeling of pins and needles when going to the loo. It wasn't unpleasant, and I dismissed it as just another of those oddities of growing old. Some time later, when I was reaching up and fiddling with a dodgy curtain track, I experienced the same sensation. I did some lateral thinking and came to the conclusion it was caused by the angle of my head, perhaps tipping my head back compressed some nerve. When I sit on the loo I lean forward, elbows on knees and look up. So, if gentlemen look down, ladies look up. It ain't what you do, it's the way that you do it! But either way can give you a tingle.'

♦ Retired physician Dr R.G. Willison from Oxford is not convinced. 'I find it hard to believe this is anything to do with neck posture. I remember discussing the phenomenon at the Department of Anatomy at Oxford when I was a student. My neck was in rather better shape than it is today. I have noticed it on and off over the years. I would describe the sensation as a warm, slightly painful tingling in the palms of the hands. It lasts a couple of seconds and ceases as soon as the urine flows.'

URINARY BLEEDING AND PAIN

The combination of excruciating pain in one or other flank, followed by red-stained urine due to the presence of blood can mean only one thing – the presence of a kidney stone being passed down the ureter into the bladder. There is usually no difficulty making the diagnosis with an X-ray of the kidney and appropriate tests. Sometimes, however, there is nothing to be found, and the questions arises as to what might be causing these symptoms. This syndrome has a name: loin pain/ haematuria (blood in the urine) syndrome.

Query 41-year-old Mrs N.B. from Devon writes:

About two years ago at a routine medical examination I was found to have *large amounts of blood in my urine*. My family doctor could find no obvious cause and referred me to the relevant specialists, who after completing many tests, put it down to being just one of those things. The bleeding continued without any physical symptoms until six months ago, when I began to experience *extreme pain in the lower right-hand side of my abdomen*. At the same time I began to pass occasional blood clots varying in size from a pinhead to about a third of the size of a golf ball! The pain is severe enough to cause me to stream with sweat and according to my husband I also become very pale. It almost always occurs in the evenings, physical activity – even gentle walks – usually precede the onset of pain. My consultant says the pain 'is entirely consistent with renal colic', but despite having repeated all the previous tests, they have been unable to find any abnormality.

I have been advised to try acupuncture (which is not helping) but apart from that the consultants admit they are baffled and I have been left to 'await further developments' – assuming there are some. Meanwhile my sex life has ceased, I have given up my hobbies (golf, swimming, walking, etc.) because they are too painful. My job is at risk, I have no social life and I am finding driving difficult either due to extreme pain or the effects of painkillers.

Comment The loin pain/haematuria syndrome was first described in 1967 in three women in whom, despite the most thorough investigations, no cause was found for their pain and bleeding. The cause remains obscure though there is a suggestion that it might be related to the blood supply to the kidney. Dr R.P. Burden from Portsmouth writes: 'The syndrome is characterized by repeated attacks of unilateral or bilateral severe loin pain, severe loin tenderness and often – but not invariably – haematuria. We believe the syndrome is more common than is generally realized and symptoms are often wrongly ascribed to urinary infections or to skeletal or gynaecological or even neurotic origins.'

Treatment

(i) *Strong analgesics*: The severity of the pain is such that many require strong opiate drugs such as morphine.

(ii) *Capsaicin*: Capsaicin is derived from chilli peppers. It vigorously stimulates the nerve fibres, thus depleting them of the neurotransmitter chemical which is involved in the experience of pain and so desensitizing the nerve. The technique involves instilling a solution of Capsaicin into the lower part of the ureter. Dr T. Armstrong from Hampshire reports that six out of ten patients who received the treatment obtained 'short- to medium-term' symptomatic relief, and in four it had no effect.

(iii) *Gabapentin*: Gabapentin – originally introduced as an anti-epileptic drug – has an important role in the treatment of syndromes associated with pain, presumably by 'dampening down' the firing of the relevant pain fibres. Fifty-six year-old Mrs J.A. from Hampshire describes her experience with these two treatments and the problems that patients can encounter.

> I have suffered from this condition for the last six years. In my case the pain is on the left side and starts in my back and comes through in waves to the lower front of my abdomen. They have been described as classic renal colic and is certainly the most severe pain I have ever had – including childbirth. Investigations show the pain was accompanied by haematuria, but I have never passed blood clots. After a couple of years of X-rays, scans and kidney function tests, no cause was found. My consultant was conducting trials for the use of Capsaicin for this syndrome. Assuming the alternative was the prospect of a lifetime on morphine I agreed to take part. A solution of Capsaicin was instilled into my left ureter under anaesthetic and the theory was that it overloaded the nerve fibres concerned so they stopped registering pain. To my delight it worked and I was pain free for the best part of a year.
>
> I was told that if the effect of the treatment wore off, the treatment could be repeated but during my pain-free year it was announced the hospital was to close and many staff, including the consultant, moved elsewhere. When my pain did return, the new consultant was opposed to this treatment on the grounds that it would 'kill my kidney' and instead he referred me to the pain clinic, where I went back to my previous state of surviving on morphine. We started on Gabapentin which, to my astonishment, worked, but the downside was I felt muzzy and sleepy all the time. Then I was given *carte blanche* to increase or decrease the dose

according to how I was and I have managed to spend most of the time on a low enough dose to feel almost normal. My outlook now is I have to live with this for the rest of my life.

(iv) *Kidney autotransplantation*: This rather drastic procedure involves transferring the kidney from its normal position down into the groin, in the process of which it loses its nerve supply but preserves its function. An editorial in *The Lancet* observed: 'Autotransplantation may seem a desperate treatment for a syndrome that does not lead to loss of kidney function, but the operation may save patients' repeated attacks of pain requiring heavy analgesia.'

FREQUENT NOCTURNAL URINATION (NOCTURNAL POLYURIA)

Query 1 74-year-old former medical secretary Mrs D.A. from Surrey writes: 'I am fortunately agile enough *to get out of bed seven or eight times a night to pass large volumes of urine – no matter if I have a late drink or not*. In between these perambulations I always have restless sleep with vivid dreams, often looking desperately for a ladies room.'

Query 2 79-year-old Mrs G.C. from Jersey writes:

For some years now I have had to get up four or five times a night. My family doctor suggested sleeping pills, but one still has to get up to urinate, so I just get on with it. Listening to the World Service, watching a little TV, walking in the garden and having a spoonful of yoghurt. Then after 15–20 minutes, return to sleep (thankfully without nightmares) until the next interruption. Compared with the problems many people have to endure, I feel watching the stars, hearing the dawn chorus and the World Service is not so bad.

Comment There are several conditions where sleep is disturbed by the requirement to rise and pass urine at night, such as bladder infections, interstitial cystitis, an enlarged prostate and problems with bladder muscle function. These correspondents, however, note the passage of *large quantities* of urine in the absence of an underlying bladder problem. This has a name, nocturnal polyuria syndrome (NPS) – literally passing a lot of urine at night – and is due to an age-related disturbance of the secretion of the hormone ADH, or antidiuretic hormone, which, as its name suggests, prevents or reduces diuresis or the production of urine. There is a cyclical rhythm of ADH secretion over a period of 24 hours, being maximal at night, which is why it is usually not necessary to rise at night, except for those who have had several pints in the pub that evening. This cyclical rhythm is presumed to be disrupted in those with NPS.

Treatment

(i) *Desmopressin*: Those who produce no ADH at all have the condition diabetes insipidus and produce large quantities of urine over 24 hours. This is corrected by nasal inhalation of a drug with the same chemical structure, desmopressin. This is obviously also an option for those with nocturnal polyuria syndrome, where the problem rather is a relative lack of ADH at night when it is most needed.

> My problem has been alleviated by the inhalation of Desmopressin nasal spray before retiring to bed. It has certainly revolutionized my life, as I now have to wander to the toilet only twice each night (occasionally not at all) which means I have a greatly improved sleeping pattern. My husband often comments he doesn't see why putting something up my nose should stop me peeing! Frankly I don't care. I am just relieved to be rid of the predicament.

Desmopressin can, however, raise the blood pressure, so cannot be prescribed to those over 65 and those most likely to suffer from this condition. Therefore alternative possibilities must also be considered.

(ii) *Red wine*: 'I find the answer is red wine with supper – in fact the more the better. Quite independently a friend has found the same happy remedy. White wine does not have the same effect, so what is the difference? Tanin perhaps.'

(iii) *Positive thinking*:

> My aged parents in their 80s retire to their bedroom at night with a bedchamber pot just under their bed. They make use of it during the night without undue perambulations down the corridor. If your reader wants to do the same and on retiring say to herself 'I do not need to find a ladies room, I am already in one,' it would in theory and, hopefully in practice, pre-empt the need to find one in her dreams. I suspect this would have to be said and done regularly every night until the change in pattern from her present situation becomes effective.

(iv) *Diuretics*: 'I also have disturbed sleep with dreams involving a search for a loo, which only stopped when I eventually wake and got out of bed. My doctor recently prescribed the diuretic Frusemide – taken at teatime. During the next three or four hours I urinate frequently, but have not had to get up in the night since.'

(v) *Aspirin*: Aspirin and related non-steroidal anti-inflammatory drugs such as Indomethacin and Ibuprofen block a hormone that regulates the flow of blood to the kidneys, thus reducing the amount of urine produced. Indomethacin is used in various kidney conditions associated with excess urine, but the value of this class of drugs in the treatment of NPS was first identified, by chance, by Dr Eric Lewis of Weston-super-Mare.

> I have suffered from this annoying complaint for several years passing up to one and a half litres overnight during four or five trips to the toilet. This despite taking no fluids after 6 p.m. I have, however, hit upon a simple remedy which I hope will work for your readers as well as it does for me. 600mg of soluble aspirin in half a glass of water taken before I go to bed reduces my need to rise to once at most and blissfully allows me to sleep until 7 a.m. – rather than being forced out of bed at 5.30 a.m. with a bursting bladder never to get back to sleep.

Twelve readers subsequently wrote to report a similar response, with a mean reduction in nocturnal frequency from 4.2 to 0.8 times per night. Seven had been prompted to try aspirin having read the article, and a further five (one with

aspirin, two with Ibuprofen and two Diclofenac) had independently noticed the effect, suggesting it is common to this
class of drug.

BURNING BLADDER PAIN (INTERSTITIAL CYSTITIS)

Interstitial cystitis is one of several ailments that closely mimic
some other straightforward medical condition – in this case the
bladder infection cystitis. The symptoms of pain on urination
and increased frequency are the same, but when the doctors
perform their investigations, take biopsies, do blood tests and
swabs, there is no evidence of infection.

Query 1 78-year-old retired secretary Mrs P.I. from Newbury
writes:

> I have had *irritable bladder syndrome for over ten years due to
> retention of urine and acidity.* I follow all the usual preventative
> and remedial methods such as avoiding citrus fruits etc., paying
> scrupulous attention to hygiene – you name it, I've tried them all!
> The pain is very wearisome and I can't stay far from a loo since I
> have to 'go' every hour. My doctor is at a loss with my problem
> so I am feeling rather forlorn.

Query 2 Mrs S.D., writing on behalf of her daughter Charlotte, writes:

> Charlotte was always a very bright sunny girl who achieved well
> at everything, always very conscientious, she was at the top of the
> form and showed much promise musically and artistically. She first
> consulted her doctor at the age of 18 with a bad attack of cystitis,
> since when she has suffered from it on a more or less permanent
> basis. *She is in pain for most of the time, describing it as though
> her lower body is on fire,* is afraid to spend a penny and at the
> same time afraid to put it off, knowing it only makes it worse. The
> pain she describes as 'peeing razor blades'. She has been referred
> to many specialists, who always begin by assuring her they can
> help. She has had various investigative operations. She starts full
> of hope, but it always ends in despair. She has tried nutritionists,
> acupuncturists, massage, really everything. Recently her family

doctor suggested her symptoms were likely to persist 'for ever' and she should concentrate on coping with the pain. She is certainly unhappy a lot of the time. Everything is a struggle, her career, social life and, needless to say, with this particular pain, any intimate personal relationship. She is surrounded by a loving family who are all helpless as we watch this vibrant spirit being broken.

Comment The lining of the bladder appears inflamed in patients with interstitial cystitis, though by definition its cause is not known. Various possible explanations have included toxic substances in the urine, the loss of protective lining of the inner bladder wall, several 'undetectable' infective agents and disturbance of nerve function. The range of treatments – as always when none is particularly satisfactory – are legion. We start with the simple ones:

Identify food allergy/sensitivity Many people report that their symptoms are precipitated or exacerbated by a variety of different foods, of which the main culprits are *acidic fruits and tomatoes*.

- ◆ 'It took me three years to find out the problem was acid of any kind: citrus juice, wine, brandy, sherry and gin and tonic (but thank goodness not beer or whisky), vinegar, most fruits and even marmalade. The reason it took me so long was that the various items took differing times to affect the bladder; for instance it was 36 hours after drinking wine before it affected me and it took three days to clear through; orange juice reacted almost immediately but the effect was over within hours; vinegar came somewhere in the middle. I took my story to my current doctor but it was obvious he didn't believe me and it was a great relief to find another sufferer – believe it or not – at a cocktail party. I was able to believe I wasn't imagining 15 years of misery (walking downstairs was uncomfortable, a car ride was awful and sex was hell!)'
- ◆ *Chocolate*: 'I was told to give up caffeine. In the event this has turned out to mean chocolate as well as tea and

coffee. This has been an adjustment and combined with taking generous amounts of water has sorted out the problem.'

♦ *Milk products*: 'Ten years ago aged 40 I underwent countless tests and courses of antibiotics only to be told nothing was wrong. Desperate for help I consulted the medical herbalist, who diagnosed an intolerance to lactose. If I avoid all milk products I am totally free of the symptoms.'

♦ *Sugar*: If I keep off refined sugar and avoid too much fruit I remain pain free and out of the bathroom. One slice of very ripe melon is enough to bring back the pain.

♦ *Food additives*: 'In desperation I went to see a doctor who specializes in complementary medicine, who had some wonderful equipment that identifies whether you are allergic to to any particular food or chemicals. I was diagnosed as being allergic to benzoic acid and by avoiding foods containing this I saw a dramatic improvement within a week.'

♦ *Carbonated drinks*: 'Several years ago I suffered cystitis for three summers running. The doctor could find no trace of infection. Finally I realized the cause of this myself. I worked for a soft drinks manufacturing company and soft drinks were available to all employees. Although I do not normally drink squash or carbonated drinks I was tempted to during the summer months and together with the rest of the girls in the office I drank diet carbonated drinks. During the third summer I realized the onset of cystitis symptoms coincided with this habit and so I stopped and the symptoms promptly disappeared. Recently I bought a bottle of diet blackcurrant squash and immediately the symptoms appeared again. I presume my bladder is sensitive to to an ingredient used in these drinks.'

♦ *Miscellaneous*: The other food group implicated in interstitial cystitis is that containing tyramine, which is wine, cheese, beer, pickled herrings, avocados, certain cheeses, nuts and soy sauce.

Those wishing to self-experiment to find which, if any, foods or drinks might be responsible, should follow the following procedure:

♦ Fast for five days, drinking only filtered water. If the symptoms don't improve during the fast, the trouble is not food allergy, but if they do improve you should introduce one food or drink on the sixth day. (If the food is an allergen, the consequence will, in their unmasked state, be dire. Sodium bicarbonate can be used to clear the system. Then go on introducing a new food on each succeeding day until enough safe foods have been discovered and the allergens found and discarded.

Simple Remedies

(i) *Sodium bicarbonate*: Reducing the acidity of the urine provides remarkable symptomatic relief. The method is to dissolve one spoonful of bicarbonate of soda in half a pint of water and drink as many half pints of this as possible. As soon as the mixture hits the bladder, relief ensues. This can be supplemented a few hours later by taking four Tums or another form of calcium carbonate. This will slowly release bicarbonate into the bladder.

(ii) *Cranberry juice*: Cranberry juice is widely recognized as being very effective in bacterial cystitis, though some report it exacerbates the symptoms of interstitial cystitis.

(iii) *Evening primrose oil*: 'I am either cured or in a lengthy period of remission following the chance discovery that evening primrose oil seems to be beneficial. I take cod liver oil capsules to ease my slightly rheumatic thumb joint and one day when I went to renew the supply, the only capsule available was cod liver oil with evening primrose oil so I decided they wouldn't do me any harm and bought them. About two days later I realised my trips to the bathroom were much less frequent and the constant slight pain had eased. That was a year ago and I have been well ever since. Instead of three or four visits to the bathroom in the night I now only have to get up once. I cannot begin to describe the joy of having four or five hours of uninterrupted sleep after all those years of disturbed nights.'

(iv) *Homeopathy*: 'The homeopathic treatment that really helped was a course of cantharis. I now get out of bed just twice and the burning sensation isn't nearly as intense. Also I have discovered a mug of camomile tea after the last meal of the day can help.'

(v) *Bladder exercises*: 'For years I was miserable with pain and worried if I was out of sight of a toilet. Thinking there was no cure I just put up with it. Eventually I was referred to the local hospital and this is what the consultant prescribed: Try to "hold on" for one hour initially. When you have been successful for three consecutive days try to "hold on" for one and a half hours. When you have managed that for three consecutive days go to two hours, then three hours and even four hours. If you fall by the wayside, keep trying until you achieve three days at each stage. Within 6–8 weeks I was cured. If I feel similar symptoms recurring I make myself wait maybe another half hour until the very last minute. The consultant said there is no underlying infection causing the problem, it is a matter of retraining the bladder.'

Medication

(i) *Steroids and antibiotics*: The lack of a clear understanding of the cause of interstitial cystitis could mean that several different factors might be responsible for the same symptoms, thus even though there is no evidence of infection, some claim benefit from the antibiotic Furadantin while others from the strong anti-inflammatory medication steroids: 'My local family doctor prescribed after much trial and error a course of Furadantin 50mg and subsequently continued with one tablet each night without fail. This treatment has cured my symptoms and I can go about daily life with confidence after years of distress.'

(ii) *Cimetidine*: Cimetidine, the well-known treatment for peptic ulcers and gastritis, works by blocking the action of the chemical histamine in the lining of the stomach which in turn reduces the amount of acid secretion. The bladder wall in patients with interstitial cystitis contains cells with a lot of histamine, and so theoretically Cimetidine might also be of benefit in reducing pain and frequency of urination. Pieter Seshadri, urologist at Queen's University, Ontario, reports an almost 50 per cent complete and sustained response to the medication:

> I was in a shocking state. I was in dreadful discomfort because of the overwhelming need to keep going to the loo. The more I went, the worse everything became. I started bleeding and felt as though I was passing glass. I forced myself to go only when my bladder was really full. I wasn't able to sleep or function properly and sex was definitely on hold. I was able to continue working because my family was very supportive. Following several months' treatment with Cimetidine I noticed I was gradually getting better. Now I am back to normal and can wear jeans and ride my motorbike which would have been agony when I was ill.

(iii) *Gabapentin*: The anti-epileptic drug Gabapentin is reputed to reduce the pain in a similar way as it works in epilepsy, by damping down the action of the nerve fibres. Dr Hans Henson reports the following case history:

> A 28-year-old woman was referred by a urologist for management of her pain caused by her interstitial cystitis. Her activities of daily living were impaired by the pain and she was not working. Gabapentin was initiated at 300mg three times a day and after six weeks of therapy she noticed 'enhanced restorative sleep', decreased use of analgesics and better function in daily activities. She is contemplating returning to work and is pleased with the tolerance level and minimal side-effects of the drug.

12

Legs and Feet

The legs and feet are a biomechanical marvel, both sustaining the weight of the human frame while providing forward propulsion. The misfortunes that befall them are predictable enough. The burden of sustaining such pressures over many years erodes the cartilages of the joints to cause arthritis. Alternatively, the blood vessels to these far parts of the body become narrowed, resulting in cramping pain (analagous to angina) on walking, due to insufficient blood supply to the leg muscles.

These and other age-related problems are usually quite straightforward, but the syndromes described here are amongst the most bizarre of all medical conditions.

RESTLESS LEGS

The restlessness of restless legs is driven by a most peculiar creeping or crawling sensation in the legs while at rest, which can only be relieved by movement. The Swedish physician K.A. Ekbom first described the condition back in 1960:

> Graphic descriptions are sometimes heard such as '*it feels as if my whole leg is full of small worms,*' or '*as if ants are running up and down my bones,*' or '*it feels like an internal itch.*' They are all agreed on two points: first, that as long as the sensations last, *it is impossible to keep their legs still*, and second that the condition is exceedingly unpleasant. 'It is a diabolical feeling,' 'I would not wish it on my worst enemy,' 'It spoils my whole life,' 'severe

creeping sensations can produce general irritation or despair,' 'I get so angry that I swear.' An otherwise well-balanced hospital nurse said 'I get so hysterical that I weep.'

In the daytime the discomfort may disappear completely, but it often starts when the patients have to sit still for any length of time, especially in the evening, when they are tired. The sensations are worse on trains, journeys and at lectures, the theatre and cinema. Some say they can never have a moment's peace. They can never sink into an armchair and relax. They cannot sit still at a bridge table or dinner party. Their discomforts force them to walk up and down constantly 'like a lost soul'. Disregarding the creeping sensations during the daytime is only a minor discomfort. They do not become unbearable until it is time for bed.

The creeping sensation starts a short time after getting into bed. In the severest cases they persist with interruptions until three, four or five in the morning. When the sensation starts it is impossible to keep the legs still. They lie kicking or moving their legs around or massaging them. They often have to get up and walk. 'Like a caged bear, they sit and smoke, knit, read or play patience, kicking all the time.' After a time ranging from a few minutes to an hour the creeping sensation ceases and the patient returns to bed. He may fall asleep, often, however, the sensations reappear after an interval and the same cycle may be repeated many times during the night.

Close examination of sufferers reveals no abnormality; nor do other investigatory tests. No abnormalities of muscles or nerves have ever been identified, though as will be seen, the cause is presumed to lie deep in the sensory part of the brain.

Treatment There are now some very effective drugs for restless legs, but the following manoeuvres have also been reported to be helpful.

(i) *Heat*: Heat in the form of a hot bath last thing at night or a hot water bottle and cold socks can prevent restless legs. Blessed relief is sometimes reported during a viral illness such as flu which, by raising the temperature, provides relief for a few days.

(ii) *Cold*: Alternatively, some find relief by pouring icy water over their legs. Lying horizontal on the ground and sticking their feet into the refrigerator or, weather permitting, walking bare foot in the snow. A doctor from North London writes: 'I remove all the bedding from my legs and allow them to cool. After about 30 minutes the sensation of restless legs subsides and I can cover up and go to sleep.'

(iii) *Exercise*: Lie on the floor and 'cycle' in the air until the muscles ease up.

(iv) *Cramp*: Interestingly, deliberately inducing an attack of cramp can bring relief:

> Having been driven up the wall (literally) with restless legs and tried everything, eventually out of desperation I pulled my calf muscles so tight that very quickly I got cramp in the leg. Letting go, I immediately noticed this infernal irritation had just about disappeared. Now when I feel the restless legs about to start up, I induce a cramp, let go immediately and have no more trouble. Sometimes I have to repeat the process a few times but no more.

(v) *Iron*: For some reason restless legs is exacerbated by anaemia due to lack of iron and will be ameliorated by its replacement.

Drugs The medical breakthrough in the treatment of restless legs came with the investigation of a man with a hereditary form of the condition.

> All his life, this 36-year-old man had unpleasant creeping sensations in both legs that kept him from falling asleep at night. The onset of these problems was traced to infancy when his mother had observed the repetitive leg movements. Eight other members of his family were affected, in all of whom symptoms began in the first year of life. They all complained of an irresistible urge that moves the legs while at rest.

A physician, Dr J. Montplaisir from Quebec, performed a lumbar puncture which revealed a very high level of the neurotransmitter dopamine in the cerebro-spinal fluid. This he speculated must be the cause, and for which the obvious treatment was to take a drug that antagonized its effect. Paradoxically this had the reverse effect to that which was anticipated, making the restless legs much worse. Dr Montplaisir then did the obvious thing and gave his patient the well-known Parkinson's drug for *increasing* the amount of dopamine in the brain – L-dopa – with the beneficial result that his restless legs completely disappeared. This, however, proved something of a false dawn, as after a few months of treatment the symptoms returned. Since then several other drugs have been found to be effective, of which the most favoured are Ropinirole and Clonazepam.

> For 14 years a 24-year-old man had experienced severe discomfort in the legs when trying to relax in the evening. On going to bed sensations would increase and spread to the arms and shoulders. They could be momentarily relieved by moving the limbs but often he would have to rise from his bed and walk around the house. When the discomfort was particularly severe it would be accompanied by involuntary jerking of the legs, which according to his wife, would continue for several hours during sleep. Clonazepam 1mg given an hour before retiring immediately and completely abolished his nocturnal symptoms. Relief has been maintained by continuing this dose without side effects.

JUMPING LEGS

There are two main types of jumping legs syndrome – periodic leg movement and sudden body jerks.

Periodic Leg Movements (Nocturnal Myoclonus)

This is closely related to restless legs, as they often (if not invariably) occur together. They have been described as follows:

> Period leg movements during sleep and relaxed wakefulness are *highly regular, jerky movements characterized by involuntary repetitive extensions of the big toe*, often accompanied by flexions of the hip, knees and ankles. Patients may not be aware of their movements but often their bed partners find they are kicked during the night.

Treatment The range of treatment is similar to that for restless legs, with Clonazepam being the most favoured. Dr Ron Pered from Haifa comments:

> Clonazepam was found to be very effective both by subjective and objective criteria. It significantly decreased the number of leg movements per hour of sleep particularly in leg movements followed by arousal, and improved sleep. Dosage adjustment is crucial. Each patient warrants individual dose adjustment, since insufficient medication is ineffective, and excessive may cause exacerbation of daytime tiredness and drowsiness.

Sudden Body Jerks

The second type of jumping legs is much commoner and Ian Oswald, psychologist at Oxford University, found on enquiring that 25 out of 50 of his acquaintances reported experiencing them up to three times a year. They may range in severity from the odd spasm to a much more violent jerk as described by 80-year-old Mr W.H. from Essex:

> I am conscious of the onset for a short while before, when I have the sensation always in my left knee of interior heat followed by an ache. *Often the jerks are considerable, lifting my leg as much as a foot above the mattress.* Most of the jerks take place in the left leg though much less frequently they start in the right. Just now and then I get the jerks when sitting in a chair which I attribute to pressure on the rear thigh and knee. Hanging on to either sides gives no relief.

Dr Oswald describes a similar case in a 32-year-old man.

> The jerks have become frequent in the previous three years, occuring three to four nights a week and as often as every couple of minutes, and might prevent him from getting to sleep for an hour or two. He had relative periods of freedom lasting weeks at a time. He thought an evening drink of beer reduced their frequency. He described the jerks as being accompanied by a feeling of flow or 'hot' quality down one or both legs. When this reached the foot or feet, a jerk occurred, then a feeling of 'swelling' shot up through his body to his head, which seemed to swell right out. He was

adamant these jerks occurred when he was still awake. When in bed he would indulge in various antics, such as sticking his legs straight up in the air in order to prevent the jerks. His performances troubled his wife.

PAINFUL LEGS AND WRIGGLING TOES

This is amongst the most grievous and bizarre of all mystery syndromes. Dr J.D. Spillane from Cardiff describes a classic case:

> A 48-year-old man was seen at Cardiff Royal Infirmary with pain in his legs for one year. *On the right the pain was only slight and came on only occasionally. On the left the pain was 'burning, throbbing, as if the leg was going to burst', and 'crushing'.* Within a few minutes of this onset, the pain was preventing sleep. The patient would go out for a walk at night to try to tire himself enough so he would fall asleep. He also had writhing movements of the left fourth and fifth toes. Over the next few years the pain never ceased and the patient lost weight and insomnia was severe. It was like 'being crushed and being on fire'. For a few minutes he would get relief by putting the leg in cold water. It was made worse by walking and was not relieved by rest. He was obviously depressed. The movements of the toes continued: purposeless, fanning, clawing and writhing.

Treatment Regrettably there is no really satisfactory treatment, though relief can be obtained with a combination of the drugs Baclofen and Clonazepam.

BURNING FEET

The sensation of burning feet in bed and night is a common – and very distressing – symptom. There are quite two distinct causes.

Query 1 74-year-old retired photographer Mr S.P. from Surrey writes:

> I have burning foot syndrome, a *mixture of pain and burning sensation on the soles of both feet.* I get good relief when standing

and therefore putting the weight of my body on the feet so there is not much of a problem during the day. The main trouble is at night where the pain either stops me from going to sleep properly or wakes me up every couple of hours. So now I have insomnia, or at any rate difficulty in sleeping. It has become most troublesome.

Query 2 78-year-old Dr T.O. from Bideford writes: 'For the last few years I have had burning in both feet, mainly in the evenings, sitting in a chair watching the television and in bed during the first half of the night. Relief is obtained by standing and walking about, but this is short-lived and acts like a counter-irritant. My feet are pinker when they "burn".'

Comment These two queries illustrate the two quite different causes of burning feet. The first Mr S.P., is due to an abnormality of the sensory nerves to the legs (or neuropathy) whereas Dr T.O. – who has the additional symptom of associated pinkness of the feet – has the skin condition known as erythromelalgia. They will be considered separately.

Neuropathy

For most, the symptom of burning feet is a sign of age – the relevant sensory nerves of the legs are just not working as well as they once were. It may, however, also be a symptom of some other illness in which the nerves are damaged, such as vitamin deficiency or diabetes.

♦ *Vitamin deficiency*: Severe malnourishment associated with vitamin deficiency is a cause of burning feet. The famous Australian doctor 'Weary' Dunlop, who as a Japanese prisoner of war worked on the notorious Thai Burma death railway, noted in his diary: 'The health of the troops is of considerable worry – over a third of them look quite ill, thin, pale and drawn. Nearly everyone is underweight with haggard, lined faces. Burning feet is one source of terrible discomfort, the feet being most exquisitely sensitive and sleep and rest are being lost.' The symptoms can persist long after malnutrition is corrected as Dr Geoffrey Gill of Liverpool School of Tropical Medicine describes: 'A 57-year-old former Far Eastern prisoner of war had been interned in Rangoon during the war where he suffered chronic dysentry and lost 32 kilos in weight. He developed burning of the hands and legs, unsteadiness in the dark, deafness and poor vision. After the war his symptoms gradually improved, but the unsteadiness and burning feet persisted. He was regularly kept awake at night by the pain and had to walk around the house to gain relief.'

♦ *Diabetes*: Diabetes is much the commonest cause of neuropathy and so diabetics are particularly prone to burning feet. Occasionally it may indeed be the first symptoms of the condition preceding the usual complaint of excess thirst and weight loss: 'When I had burning feet, a blood test showed I had late onset diabetes. I found cutting sugar out of my diet brought about an almost immediate improvement.'

♦ *Spinal problems*: Trauma or other abnormalities of the spine by interfering with the nerve fibre signals from the feet may also be responsible. 'Following a back injury 30 years ago I have a loss of sensation over a considerable surface area of the legs and feet. Besides burning feet I also get stabbing pains and intense tingling sensations – which are worse at night.'

♦ *Neck arthritis*: Those with arthritis of the upper cervical spine flexing the neck can induce a burning sensation in the feet due – presumably – to pressure on the relative nerves: 'If I ever look down – even from steep stairs – the soles of my feet burn. I once went up a funicular railway and had to be carried off – the pain was so excruciating. It was awful. I just can't – and daren't – look down if I wish to keep mobile.'

Treatment Those with diabetes should clearly ensure that their blood sugar is well controlled and there are some reports that even in the absence of vitamin deficiency, supplements are of help.

I read an article which described how some sufferers could be helped with pantothenic acid combined with magnesium. I do the same and my 'hot foot' syndrome disappeared altogether. After a few weeks I stopped the treatment and the problem recurred. So it does work.

The other options are either to apply some cooling or soothing balm to the legs or medication.

Cold and other remedies

(i) Dr Peter Dyck of the Mayo Clinic reports: 'A 65-year-old farmer had had burning soles of the feet for most of his life. He would often take off his shoes and walk barefoot behind the plough in the cool furrow to obtain relief. Before going to bed he would sit with his feet in cold water from the well or in ice water.'

(ii) 'I too suffer from hot painful feet at night. The only answer seems to be a cold hot water bottle kept inside the bed covers but away from the body, i.e. tucked at the side of the bed until needed. When the heat and pain being to rise, put the feet on the cold hot water bottle which will cool the feet and the pain will go as well.'

(iii) 'I find some relief is obtained by applying a simple foot balm such as Valpeda or ultra cooling gel.'

(iv) 'I wake in bed with a burning heel. I keep beside my bed Rhuss tox cream sold by Boots in the herbal section. I put some cream on my heel and the trouble stops.'

Medication The therapeutic options – as for all chronic pain syndromes – are either low dose antidepressants (Amitryptilene) or anti-epileptic drugs (Clonazepam), which alter the conduction of signals through the nerve fibres. The anti-Parkinson's drug L-dopa is also claimed to be 'promising':

> Burning feet has caused me many broken nights – walking on a stone floor or in summer on the dewy grass, sometimes three times a night. I slept with my feet uncovered to the despair of the medical staff during hospitalisation several times for unrelated conditions. However, some years ago my family doctor prescribed Clonazepam which he had read about in *The Lancet* and from

which he had learnt that though usually prescribed for epilepsy, a side-effect appeared to be a cure for burning feet.

Erythromelalgia

The appearance of a red or pink discoloration of the feet indicates dilation of the blood vessels and is strongly suggestive of the alternative diagnosis for burning feet of erythromelalgia, first described by an American neurologist (and best selling novelist) Silas Weir Mitchell. The cause is not known.

Treatment The soothing treatment is similar to that for neuropathic burning foot syndrome, but the medication is very different.

(i) Regular contrast foot bathing is helpful: one minute hot water, ten seconds with cold, alternating five times.
(ii) 'I find relief is achieved by dissipating body heat in other ways. So when the feet start to burn, instead of taking off your socks, take off your cardigan or pullover, remove your tie, open up the neck so that heat can be lost from the upper chest. In bed, throw out the hot water bottle, remove a blanket and even your pyjamas. Even after 15 or 30 minutes it slowly dawns on you that you are no longer conscious of your feet.'

Medication The underlying problem is dilation of the blood vessels, and thus theoretically drugs that constrict them, such as beta blockers or those used in the treatment of migraine should be of help.

A 48-year-old woman has had severe frequent crises of burning feelings accompanied by redness of both feet and ankles for ten years. These crises were precipitated by heat and were much worse in summer and in bed at night, and she needed to put both feet in cold water with ice several times a day and night. The condition has been worse for the past year and she had to sleep with her feet wrapped in wet towels, walk bare foot and keep a pool of cold water nearby at her workplace. Her life was becoming unbearable. I tried Propranolol 10mg three times a day. The result was dramatic from the outset and for the past few months she has been free of symptoms. The response to the anti-migraine drug Pizotifen has also been reported as being 'spectacular'.

ITCHY FEET

Query 71-year-old senior manager Mr C.K. from Nottingham writes:

> My problem, for the last ten years, is a *deep-seated and painful 'itch' which affects my sleep*. The complaint happens usually at night and can affect one or both feet, usually the soles but sometimes the side of the foot. It is painful enough to waken me and keep me awake. My excellent family doctor has prescribed antihistamine creams. I have also used witch hazel gel – both afford some relief but slowly. They do not seem very effective.

Comment There are of course many causes of itchy feet, but here the close similarity with burning feet – the symptoms being worse at night and relieved by walking about – strongly suggest that this is a variant of the neuropathic form of the syndrome. It was not, however, possible to find any previous account of this 'itchy foot syndrome', though one correspondent observed that it was the presenting sign of her daughter's Hodgkin's disease: 'My daughter had an itch on both her feet which was severe and kept her awake at night. We went from doctor to doctor, no one could help, they just gave her cream and oil. She was eventually seen by a skin specialist who sent her to hospital where she was diagnosed as having Hodgkin's disease.'

Treatment Massaging with moisturizing lavender foot cream and Venal (which contains horse chestnut extract) are reported to be helpful. It would be interesting to investigate whether drugs used for the treatment of restless legs might be effective in this condition.

LIGHTNING FEET PAINS

Query Mrs G.F. from Surrey writes:

> I *experience spasms of really agonising pain in one or other of my*

feet, never both at the same time. The spasms last for about five seconds, and at their worst recur every 20 seconds. They slacken off to one every few minutes then at wider intervals before easing altogether. The longest period during which the pains have occurred is 24 hours, the shortest is half an hour or less. The pains are sometimes like fork lightning, running all through my foot; sometimes like a needle being pushed into a toe; sometimes a deep stabbing pain. They are not cramp, sciatica or pins and needles. I would compare the level of pain to a dentist drilling on a nerve on a tooth. It is seriously bad.

Comment This and similar foot complaints are, like neuropathic burning foot, probably due to abnormalities of conduction of the sensory nerves in the feet.

♦ 'I experienced absolutely excruciating pain like a swarm of bees all stinging at one time on the ankle.'
♦ 'I was woken in the early hours by excruciating pain in the left ankle. The pain seemed to come in waves and lasted possibly three to four minutes. Having gone back to sleep, I was woken again with a similar pain in the right ankle – if anything more severe – in fact it was the worst pain I can recall experiencing.'

There are three possible explanations:

(i) *Diabetes*: These lightning pains are not uncommon in diabetics in whom, as with burning foot syndrome, the peripheral nerves to the feet are damaged. Treatment requires appropriate control of the blood sugar and, where appropriate, similar drugs to those described for neuropathic burning foot can be tried.

(ii) *Tarsal tunnel syndrome* The nerves to the feet pass underneath and may be compressed by a sheet of tissue known as the tarsal tunnel, comparable to the carpal tunnel in the hands, which may result in the lightning pains. Retired family doctor, Dr Alan Harrison, writes:

A few weeks ago I started to experience severe lightning pains in the soles of both feet. I had noticed a mild sensory loss on the underside of the toes for over a year before this but did nothing about it. I was referred to a neurologist and, by then, had a sensation of walking on cotton wool, even by day. This confirmed my suspicion that my problem was that of a tarsal tunnel syndrome, which he thought could be controlled by appropriate medication. If relief was not sufficient, decompression surgery – as in carpal tunnel syndrome – could be arranged.

(iii) *'Phantom' pains* These lightning pains can, it would seem, originate in the brain as they may be present even following amputation. 'The pain is unpredictable at any time during the day and night. It is so severe that normal living is impossible during an attack. I subsequently had my lower leg amputated – due to a vascular condition – but even this has not cured the condition. I still get exactly the same pain in my missing foot!'

FOOT PAIN ON WALKING

The phenomenal pressures exerted on both feet by the weight of the human frame result inevitably in a whole variety of disorders of the small bones, the joints between them and the sheet of tissue that bind them together. These are all dealt with satisfactorily by one or other of the several professional groups involved in the feet – orthopaedic surgeons, podiatrists, chiropodists and so on.

There are, however, two rather unusual pain syndromes which can take a while before they are properly diagnosed.

Morton's Neuroma

Query 1 The Rev H.B. from Shropshire writes:

Twenty or more years ago I noticed after a *ten-mile hike over rough country a slight but gradually increasing burning sensation in the second toe* – which then moved on to involve several others. Since then it usually starts in early evening, and if ignored becomes both burning and a sharp spasm of stabbing pain. During the night this can persist and at a frequency of 10–25 seconds making sleep impossible.

Query 2 Miss A.B. from Finchley writes:

> I have a *sudden quite excruciating pain in the ball of my left foot*.
> It feels like dozens of pins being stuck into me and is so severe I
> have to sit and seize my foot in my hands until it passes. It is
> definitely not cramp. It always comes at rest when I am either
> sitting or lying and it comes in attacks of about four or five
> sessions over two to three days, then I may not experience it again
> for weeks or even months.

This graphic description of stabbing pains in relation to the
cleft between the big and second toe is characteristic of a
benign nerve tumour, or Morton's neuroma, which is usually
induced by the pressure of walking, but can – as here – occur
at rest. Mr M.A. Morris, orthopaedic surgeon of the Royal
Infirmary, Salford writes: 'Patients usually complain of precisely localized pain between a pair of metatarsal heads (i.e.
between the toes) often with radiation to the toes. They
describe the pain as variously burning, shooting, knives, needles, daggers or like walking on a stone or bone. Walking or
standing precipitates the pain, while rest and especially
removal of footwear gives relief.'

Treatment

(i) *Footwear* 'My solution was to wear a Dr Scholl's foam
sleeve on my fourth toe with the aim of separating the relevant
metatarsals. This worked like a charm but if I forgot to put the
sleeve on I would again wake up with the pain. After about ten
years of this procedure I forgot one night and I had no pain
and I haven't needed to wear one since. Presumably the neuroma is regressing.'
(ii) *Operation* The obvious treatment is to remove the neuroma at operation but this is not necessarily successful, suggesting that the Morton's neuroma, though present, is not
necessarily the cause of the pain in every instance.

> About two years ago I had an operation for Morton's neuroma in
> my left foot. I presumed this would be like having a bad tooth
> removed and none of the doctors I saw ever said it might not
> work. Almost immediately after the operation I felt the same

stabbing pain and was convinced it hadn't worked. I was told this was just post-operative pain but I knew it wasn't. I had the pain at least once a day, whereas before I might go a week or so without anything happening. It is nothing to do with the shoes I am wearing, but comes on every time when I change from shoes to slippers, slippers to shoes, putting on tights or even walking in bare feet. The only way now to relieve the pain is to rub the foot starting away from the painful spot and gradually working towards the toe as it becomes less painful, and then pulling the toe out. It is all rather difficult when in a public place, e.g. a shoe shop.

Foot Pain 'First Thing in the Morning' (Plantar Fasciitis)

Query 80-year-old Mr G.H. from Kent writes:

> For the last year or more I have felt *acute pain when putting my feet to the ground*, as if all the nerve endings were uncovered. This is worse during the first hour or so after getting up in the morning – but can be actuated at any time. It is so acute I can hardly bear to cross the room even on carpets at home. It can, thank God, abate when out walking. I wear cushioned trainers and have extra thick socks, but this only helps to a limited extent.

Comment This is a condition known as plantar fasciitis – inflammation of a strong band of white glistening fibres which have an important function in maintaining the longitudinal arch of the foot, whose absence results in flat feet.

Dr Dishan Singh of the Royal Orthopaedic Hospital writes: 'The patient often gives a history of gradual onset of pain which is worst on first weight bearing in the morning; the pain becomes so incapacitating that he limps to the bathroom or hobbles around with the heel off the ground. After a few steps, the heel pain will decrease during the day but will worsen with increased activity or after a period of sitting.'

Treatment Successful treatment depends on a comprehensive programme, including heel grips, pads and supports, anti-inflammatory drugs, exercises, steroid injections and night splints.

13
Skin

The skin is the largest organ in the body and vulnerable to a whole host of unusual conditions which, even if they do not know the cause, dermatologists usually have little difficulty in diagnosing by the simple expedient of translating the appearance into Latin. Thus a rash of ever widening red circles becomes *erythema annulare centrifuguum*. Consequently there were only a handful of dermatological mysteries.

WALKER'S ANKLE RASH

Query 60-year-old retired education manager Mrs H.M. from Wiltshire writes: 'Together with several of my walking companions I noticed that after a day out on the hills I develop a *red and itchy rash around the ankle*.

Comment There were several further reports of this rash, with various suggestions as to its possible cause.

♦ *Heat rash*: 'I too suffer from walker's ankle which occurs during hot weather particularly if road walking is involved, as the heat is reflected back off the road. Also the thickness of clothing around the ankles adds to the problem. Most walkers wear two pairs of socks in their walking boots and turn the tops over. They also tend to tuck the ends of their slacks into their socks. None of this allows air to circulate.'

♦ *Pollen allergy*: 'I am an all-the-year-round walker and suffer with this problem only in summer. It seems to be much worse if I walk in shorts, and indeed on one occasion was over my calf as well as ankle. I therefore wondered if pollens and dust kicked up whilst walking might migrate into and through the socks and with perspiration set up an irritation that would take seven days or more to disappear.'

'My wife and I walk regularly in the countryside and have suffered mild instances of this rash for some years. Initially we suspected heat and resultant sweating was a cause as the problem is much worse in the summer months. It appears to us now that it is an allergy reaction, because passing through lush grassy green meadows with seeds and grass sticking in the socks seems to have the worst effect.'

♦ *Biological powders*: 'When one walks the feet swell and also sweat. I did wonder if under these conditions the fibres of the socks would be injecting residues of detergent or the silicates commonly present in household detergents.'

Treatment Mrs B.D. from Cheshire writes: 'I now take the following precautions which do seem to work.

(i) Keep the area around the lower leg/ankle cool.
(ii) Trousers rolled up slightly to allow air to circulate.
(iii) Wear loose fitting socks next to the skin.
(iv) Cotton walking socks over cotton socks, and pulled down over the boot.
(v) Apply 'Derma-Guard' solution to the skin around the ankle and lower leg.'

Further suggestions included washing socks in pure soap, rinsing well; applying a protective layer of vaseline, tea tree oil and Savlon.

There were three further mystery skin conditions, which failed to elicit any response.

PINK HANDS AND FEET

Query 85-year-old Mrs M.K. has been taking Tamoxifen for two years and writes: '*After a bath the soles of my feet are scarlet and it takes all day for it to subside.* My hands are also red, particularly first thing in the morning. I have two white arms and two pink appendages ending at the wrist, as though I had gloves on.'

BLOTCHES

Query 65-year-old Mrs C.J. from Surrey writes:

From time to time I get *blotches appearing on my upper chest, neck and around my eyes.* They look to me like blood vessels bursting or even love bites! They do not cause me any pain and though I have had this condition for almost ten years there has been no ill effect on my general health. I sometimes have to resort to wearing sunglasses when there is any sun – and scarves when it is boiling hot!

CHEEK INFECTION

Query Mrs H.M. from Devon writes:

For the last five years I have had a *mystery infection that has been travelling round the soft tissue of my cheek and has now nearly surrounded my right eye.* It has defied 20+ consultants, four intraoral operations, antibiotics by the ton, two periods of hyperbaric treatment and a year of homeopathic medicine. I have a long list of what it isn't but desperation is now looming along with plastic surgery, with no guarantee of a cure or the after-effects.

14

Puzzling Pains

Many unusual pain syndromes – in the head, face, chest, bowels and legs – are described elsewhere, but this section pursues a few more which share the common feature that they are not what they appear, but rather mimic other, better known conditions.

FINGERTIP PAIN

Query Mr D.E. from West Sussex, writing on behalf of his wife, reports:

Last year my wife thought she had a *thorn under her left thumbnail. This proved not to be the case but the tip of the thumb felt as if it was in boiling fat. The pad was very sensitive to a 'feather' touch. Strangely it could be grasped firmly without increasing the level of pain.* Visits to two of the family doctors in our practice produced neither diagnosis nor cure. A third doctor thought it might emanate from the nerves at the join of the neck and shoulder and referred the problem to a consultant neurologist. He arranged for an MRI scan, that revealed damage to the neck caused by a whiplash injury 20 years ago. He recommended physiotherapy which did no good. Our family doctor then suggested acupuncture. This was tried without any benefit. He then referred my wife to a consultant rheumatologist who said there was arthritis at the base of the thumb, but had no explanation for the original pain which was continuing unabated. She passed the problem on to the occupational therapist at the local hospital who fitted a splint. As this did no good the rheumatologist then gave two steroid injections in the base of the thumb, which gave a slight benefit, but it was only temporary. Now 18 months later the pain is as intense as ever and evidences itself in the same way, i.e. the thumb can be grasped firmly without causing additional pain but a light touch still causes a very painful burning sensation. Since the basic pain never goes away it is debilitating in the extreme. There appear to be no more avenues we can explore.

Comment Exquisite pain at the tip of the finger and under the fingernail usually arises from a benign tumour rising from glandular tissue (adenoma), fatty tissue (sebaceous cyst), blood vessels (glomus) or nerve (neuroma). They are exacerbated by pressure and relieved by an operation.

Glomus

Some 35 years ago our elder daughter aged 15 complained of a *mysteriously painful thumb* for months. We were unable to get her any successful treatment and it seemed my husband and I were the only people who believed her. In desperation we took her to an orthopaedic consultant at a London teaching hospital, who recommended surgical investigation. This revealed a glomus tumour.

Dr Wayne Shiels reports a similar case:

A 28-year-old woman experienced pain at the distal end of the left thumb for approximately eight years. It had become progressively more intense, with the area involved being exquisitely tender. An incision was made at the nail base under anaesthesia and a small light pink mass was removed which on microscopic examination proved to be a glomus tumour. Eight months later the patient was asymptomatic.

Adenoma

I have had *pain and tenderness at the base of the fingernail* of the right-hand index finger for over 25 years. The pain was worse in cold weather. I found it very painful when using a file to clean under the nail. I recall that at times I could hardly bear to play the piano as I sometimes landed on the sensitive spot. My family doctor sent me to a sceptical hand surgeon who removed part of the nail under local anaesthetic and shouted in triumph that he had 'got it', 'it' being a benign tumour of a sweat gland known as an adenoma. Since then I have had no further pain.

Regrettably Mrs D.E.'s fingernail pain was, as noted, *not* exacerbated by pressure, thus excluding a benign tumour of the nailbed such as a glomus or adenoma as a possible cause. Her pain has subsequently spread to the upper arm and left ear and remains unexplained.

NOCTURNAL HIP PAIN

Query Mrs B.D. from Hampshire writes:

> Quite suddenly for no reason ten years ago *I developed a pain in my left hip. It is worse on climbing stairs but really only hurts at night, waking me at 2.00 a.m.* I am not stiff in the morning. I have seen four specialists, three rheumatologists and one hip surgeon. I have been X-rayed and had an MRI scan, been given cortisone injections and anti-inflammatory pills. None of these have done much good although the pain is less severe than in the past. No one really knows what is going on.

Comment When hip pain is worse at night and on climbing stairs, the probable diagnosis is trochanteric bursitis – inflammation of the site (the bursa) where the muscles are inserted into the protuberant bony part of the upper leg or femur (the greater trochanter). It should respond to cortisone injections, as Dr Mohammad Shbeeb from the Mayo Clinic describes:

> A 54-year-old woman reported waxing and waning of pain in the right hip extending in to the thigh which was initially noted after climbing the stairs, but was most severe at night, especially when she attempted to lie on her right side. Localized tenderness was noted over the greater trochanter and X-rays revealed mild arthritis of the hip and scaroiliac joints. After cortisone injections she reported substantial improvement and was still free of pain six months later.

The diagnosis may not be as straightforward as it might appear, as the following account reveals:

> I had pain in my right hip when going up and down stairs and in bed at night. My hips were X-rayed and I was told they were in

excellent condition. I was therefore diagnosed as having bursitis for which I was given a deep cortisone injection. I suffer no pain at all as far as any daytime activity is concerned, but the curious thing is I still cannot lie on my right side for any length of time in bed at night or the pain comes on again. When I wake in the morning it has completely gone and I am not stiff.

Similarly, Mrs B.D.'s symptoms have persisted despite cortisone injections, thus raising the possibility that she had some condition which mimics the symptoms of trochanteric bursitis, which is labelled as pseudo-trochanteric bursitis. Dr Roger Traycoff from the Southern Illinois School of Medicine makes the following observation: 'The onset of pain in trochanteric bursitis is usually insidious and relief following cortisone injection is a major criterion confirming diagnosis. Failure to obtain relief is thus likely to be due to pseudo-trochanteric bursitis, where the pain is referred from the nerves of the lower lumbar spine, the spinal joints or ligaments. Hence treatment of the underlying cause is likely to be most effective.'

(i) 'I developed pain in my right hip on climbing stairs and when lying in bed. I thought this was due to arthritis, but an X-ray showed no damage. I had the usual injections and physiotherapy and eventually went to a chiropractor – none of which helped. An MRI scan showed a trapped nerve in my spine and I started doing spinal exercises, twisting and bending sideways and frontally. After a few days of these exercises my pain was considerably better.'

(ii) 'I had two forms of pain. The first was a dull continuous ache which was enough to wake me at night if I slept on my left side or stayed in one position too long. The second was a sharp stabbing pain as if a knife was plunged into my hip. This caused me to lurch sideways whilst gasping (and swearing) and always seemed to happen when entering smart restaurants. I had all the usual investigations which showed only mild inflammation and was told I had irritable hip syndrome, the next stop would be nerve-blocking injections in my spine under general anaesthetic. I declined. I consulted a physiotherapist who felt the pain all stemmed from my back and so I had several one-hour sessions with her followed by an hour's rehabilitation exercise. After just three or four consultations I no longer take anti-inflammatory pills and only return for a consultation if I feel my back is seizing up again.'

There were also several accounts of the benefits of the local application of heat.

(iii) 'I suffer from pain in the hip at night. The only thing I have noticed is that it mainly occurs when there is a north wind. Two friends also suffer from more pain from their arthritis when there is a north wind. Extra warmth on the painful spot helps ease the pain.'

(iv) 'I develop pain in both hips during the night, which invariably wake me at around 3.00 a.m. resulting in a very disturbed sleep. Having risen around 7.30 a.m., the hip pains disappear within an hour and I am free throughout the day. From consultations with my consultant I gather this is not arthritis. Some eight years ago I changed my orthopaedic mattress for a high quality, more yielding type and this proved satisfactory in relieving my symptoms.'

(v) 'I too have been assured my hip pain is definitely not arthritis or rheumatism. When it wakes me in the early hours of the morning my experience has been that if I can just increase the circulation of the area there is relief. The application of heat (just laying my hand over the hip can often do the trick) or a magnetic wrap usually works. If all else fails I get out of bed and move around a bit, rubbing the hip, thus improving the blood flow. This seems to bring relief and hopefully the rest of the night will be undisturbed.'

SCIATICA

There are few more clear-cut and dramatic symptoms than the powerful shooting pains down the leg caused by pressure on the sciatic nerve as it emerges from the lower back, commonly referred to as sciatica. The following case, described by Dr

Ilaria Merlo from Pavia, Italy, explains how a failure to respond to standard treatment indicates the possibility of 'an uncommon cause of a common condition'.

A 33-year-old man was referred to a hospital with an eight-year history of *right sciatic pain, exacerbated by physical activity.* He was an enthusiastic skier, trekker and soccer player and his sciatica caused him severe physical and psychological distress. He had sought several opinions and undergone numerous investigations – none of which had shown any abnormality. Neither physiotherapy nor anti-inflammatory and muscle-relaxant drugs provided any relief.

On examination he had severe pain on internal rotation of the extended leg which stretches the piriformis muscle, suggesting the diagnosis of piriformis muscle syndrome. A neurosurgeon was asked to explore the sciatic nerve and at operation there was a loop of the inferior gluteal artery compressing the sciatic nerve. Artery and nerve were carefully separated and a patch was interposed between them. Following surgery the patient's pain cleared completely. When seen a year later he had had no recurrence.

PSEUDO SHINGLES

In this instance, the pain complained of is closely similar in type and distribution to that which occurs in an attack of shingles, but there is no characteristic rash.

Query Mr R.A. from Leicestershire writes on behalf of his wife:

For the past four months my wife has been experiencing *burning sensations in her back and chest of sufficient intensity to prevent her sleeping.* The sensation started quite suddenly with burning on the left side of her back and spread to her chest/stomach. There is no redness or blisters on the skin although she had similar symptoms when she had shingles many years ago. Neither our doctor nor the various specialists she has consulted are able to explain the phenomenon.

Comment Dr Jane V. Bond comments: 'The pain suffered by Mr R.A.'s wife may well have been the result of atypical shingles leading to post-herpetic neuralgia – this apparently may develop without a preceding rash. Some years ago my sister, who lives in the United States, developed a similar severe burning pain with extreme hypersensitivity extending in a band round one side of her chest without any preceding physical signs. I persuaded her to attend the pain clinic at the Massachusetts General Hospital in Boston, where she was put through a vast number of investigations, all of which proved negative. The specialist then sent me a lengthy and detailed report, of which his final sentence reads: 'I can only conclude this patient had atypical herpes zoster and is suffering from post-herpetic neuralgia.' Once her condition had a name my sister was less anxious and the pain gradually decreased, though she still has residual hypersensitivity to touch.

Three other possibilities were suggested:

♦ *Neuralgia*: 'I have suffered the intense pain suffered by the lady quoted which started on the left lower back and then travelled round to the left hip and down into the groin. My excellent doctor admitted to being puzzled and said I should have shingles, but I did not have a rash or blisters. He therefore suspected neuralgia and sent me for some physiotherapy, concentrating on the lower back area. This took place in a hot exercise pool on a twice-weekly basis with the intention of improving the mobility and strength of my spine. This proved very successful and I have continued these exercises on a daily basis at home. The pain is gone and my back is better than it has been for years.'

♦ *Fibromyalgia*: 'I often felt the pain as a searing burning sensation and I thought a number of times it might be related to shingles. Again I had no rash. As the months wore on the pain moved round my back and neck, even sometimes round my rib cage. My GP suggested it might be fibromyalgia and the pain is being controlled by 20mg of amytriptylene, which just turns the volume of the pain down enough to be bearable.'

♦ *Relief with antihistamines*: 'It had been suggested by both the physiotherapist and an osteopath I was probably suffering from post-herpetic neuralgia, but like Mr R.A.'s wife I have never had a rash or blisters! Purely by chance I found that taking antihistamine tablets caused the symptoms to completely disappear.'

THROBBING BACK PAIN

Query Mr R.D. from Newcastle, a 65-year-old retired insurance underwriting manager, writes:

For almost a year *I have suffered from a throbbing in the kidney area when lying down.* Having emptied my bladder before going to sleep I invariably wake up after three hours with this throbbing. *Sometimes in the morning it is accompanied by feeling sick.* I have had numerous blood tests for kidney and liver function, blood sugar and cholesterol and two scans of the kidneys, bladder and gallbladder. All have proved negative – but I am still suffering!

Comment Throbbing back pain is strongly suggestive of dilation of the major artery in the abdomen – an abdominal aneurysm.

Fourteen years ago my husband had severe back pain waking him during the night. While seeking treatment from a chiropracter he could feel throbbing whilst lying face down. When he consulted his family doctor she immediately diagnosed an aortic aneurysm which was pressing on his kidneys when he lay down. He was operated on within 48 hours and has been in good health since.

Nonetheless this would not seem to be the problem in Mr R.D.'s case as the relevant investigations had excluded this possible diagnosis. Another reader whose symptoms persisted despite repair of his discovered aneurysm, suggests they were more likely to be due to some functional disturbance of the gastrointestinal tract, as his pains disappeared when he resolved not to eat for two or three hours before retiring to bed.

VAGINAL PAIN

There are several recognized – if difficult to treat – syndromes of vaginal discomfort including the itching of pruritus vulvae and the chronic pain syndromes of vulvodynia (pain in the vulva) and vestibulitis (inflammation of the vulva). Here we describe four further, all relatively treatable, causes of this distressing complaint.

'Sore Throat' Vagina

Query Mrs B.C. from Hampshire writes on behalf of a friend.

She is in her late 20s and has had this problem since she went to university at 18. Her symptoms are *a soreness in the vagina 'like a sore throat'* which is extremely painful, *a feeling of being swollen inside*, it usually *starts during the night*, begins suddenly and clears up just as suddenly, and is associated with pain on urination. All the possible causes have been eliminated by hospital tests and private and complementary treatments have all proved ineffective. The saddest consequence is this young woman avoids any emotional involvement as she is too embarrassed to explain her problem. She sees her youth and chances of romance slipping away.

Comment The following unusual if interesting solution has been suggested.

This sounds very like a problem I suffered similarly from my late teenage years and especially through my 20s. I came to the conclusion it was a peculiarly painful form of congestion. I found the solution to this problem purely by accident and it has worked ever since. It was a Pifco face massager used as a vibrator to orgasm. The congestion clears instantly and the pain vanishes. It is important it is not one of those vibrators that goes inside for the obvious reason the cure would feel worse than the problem. This was the cure I (and many other women I know) always used to brilliant effect for period cramps. All she needs to do is to buy one of these snub-nosed little electric massagers 'for a really stiff shoulder' – and a good bolt for her bedroom door.

'A Thousand Needles'

Query 68-year-old Mrs B.S. from Essex writes: '*I have a continual pricking, like a thousand needles sticking into me*

*around the vulva, vagina and extending to the back passage
and top of the leg.* It gets much worse if I am moving or
walking and has been getting more severe over the years. I find
it very distressing and painful.'

Comment A reader suggests that this may be an unusual form
of post-herpetic neuralgia.

> My mother has had a similar pain in her 'bottom' for almost eight
> years. She had every sort of scan and nerve blocks one can
> imagine. The pain is severe enough she has had codeine or varying
> strengths of morphine. She doesn't drive and socialises very little.
> She used to spend hours lying on icebags. She has been to hospitals
> in Boston and travelled to the University of Rochester Hospital for
> another, always hopeful, fine evaluation. The doctor announced he
> was 99 per cent certain it was shingles. She was given a 0.075 per
> cent Capsaicin cream and told to put it on the area four times a
> day and was told it would take eight weeks until she found
> relief.

Vaginal Pain due to Coeliac Disease

Dr Christine Costello of London's Chelsea & Westminster
Hospital describes the following case:

> A 44-year-old woman presented with a six-month history of burn-
> ing, itching and a greenish vaginal discharge. The symptoms were
> worse before and after her periods. On examination she had a
> small ulcer in the vagina, but there was nothing else of note. She
> was noted to have mild iron deficiency anaemia and further inves-
> tigations revealed a diagnosis of Coeliac disease. She was started
> on a gluten-free diet and within a few weeks her vaginal symptoms
> had markedly improved and by two months they had completely
> resolved.

Vaginal Pain due to a 'Trapped' Pudendal Nerve

Professor Ahmed Shafiq from Cairo University describes a
condition of burning vulva pain which occurs spontaneously
every two to three days and was induced by sexual intercourse.

It occurred as a 'crisis', lasting for two to four hours, which disappeared spontaneously, and was not relieved by analgesia. Examination revealed abnormality of the pudendal nerve that innervates this region. The history strongly pointed to the diagnosis of pudendal canal syndrome, and following an operation to relieve the pressure on the pudendal nerve, the pain gradually disappeared over the following four weeks.

The following three pain syndromes were also reported for which no explanations were forthcoming:

STABBING KNEE PAIN

Query Mrs L.L. from Hampshire writes:

> While walking up the garden chatting away with my daughter and husband *I experienced a sudden sharp stabbing pain at the inside of my right knee.* It was in the fleshy mound and seemed not far under the surface, was intense and lasted 25 seconds, when it stopped as suddenly as it started. Since then this same excruciating pain (always of the same intensity, lasting the same length of time and always in exactly the same place) has occurred at odd times. It doesn't seem to make any difference whether I am sitting still, standing, walking or fast asleep in bed. The most puzzling aspect is its random occurrence. Months go by without an attack, but once it starts the 25-second episodes can increase from once an hour to once every ten minutes.

CHINESE BURN

Query Mrs P.A. from Staffordshire writes:

> I am a 56-year-old woman who for the last four years has had pins and needles and *sharp stabbing pains in my hands and feet.* Over the years *these have progressed to the whole of my body, including face and scalp. The sensation is not particularly a numbness, but more a 'Chinese burn'.* Quite often I have a feeling of total exhaustion and muscle weakness that I can barely walk, and also uncomfortable bloating and swelling. Usually I have to go to bed until I recover. I wake up every morning with tingling and stabbing pains – sometimes it gets worse or better as the day goes on.

'TOTAL BODY' PINS AND NEEDLES

Query 1 Mrs J.K. from Berkshire writes:

My 70-year-old father-in-law has been afflicted by feelings of *pins and needles all over the body from head to toe* – especially arms and legs – ever since he had an angioplasty for angina. He describes it as having been in contact with nettles, with this he has a *dry mouth, sore gums and a 'rushing sound' in his ears*. The only relief he has is when he moves around. This feeling happens from the moment he wakes up and is especially worse in the evening. So far he has seen the cardiologist, dermatologist, neurologist and is now trying acupuncture. All this has had no effect whatsoever.

Query 2 Mrs M.J. from Herts writes:

It all started with pins and needles in my right shoulder. Actually it is more *as though some hot water has been poured down the shoulder.* My toes feel swollen but are not actually swollen and I continually move them about in my shoes when sitting to try and make them feel comfortable. Over the next two years the tingling sensation has progressed further up the legs and arms. I have also been getting severe pains in the legs, with a feeling of tight bands around my knees and ankles – the feeling my legs would burst. My feet are burning hot – not to touch but within themselves. Again this is always much worse at night. Then I would suddenly get two or three weeks when (apart from the tingling sensation) I would feel fine. The pains would disappear and I would feel generally much better. Then suddenly the pains and burning and feelings of ties around my knees and ankles and pressure on my legs would start again. I have had two years of investigations including being admitted to the National Neurological Hospital – all to no avail. They admit there is something wrong, but cannot find the cause.'

15
Tiredness and Fatigue: Variations on a Theme

Tiredness and fatigue are an almost universal feature of every type of illness, but tend to be overshadowed by other more specific symptoms relating to the underlying cause. However, if they occur as the sole or major symptom they can be particularly difficult to evaluate, for two fairly obvious reasons. First, tiredness and fatigue are a common symptom of depression and, secondly, even when there seems to be a problem related to some disease of nerve or muscle the mechanisms involved are obscure. Nonetheless, this section is useful in emphasizing the range of fatigue type syndromes and the various hypotheses for what might be going on.

The most useful distinction in sorting out fatigue symptoms is prising out those where the problem is primarily physical – that is related to exertion – and those in which it is both physical and mental, i.e. where there is also a sense of mental exhaustion and poor motivation.

CHRONIC FATIGUE SYNDROME

Chronic fatigue syndrome (CFS) or as it is sometimes known, ME, is both physical and mental. Its cause is unknown and has been a major source of controversy. Its main features are well recognized, but it merits discussing here because it is helpful to distinguish it from other causes of fatigue outlined below.

David Dawson, Professor of Neurology at Harvard Medical School, comments on the four distinguishing features of CFS:

♦ *Confusion, impairment of memory and difficulty in concentrating* are common. These symptoms grouped together suggest a brain disorder which is often noted to be variable. There is often trouble with arithmetic or recent and intermediate memory.

♦ Patients are described as *'emotionally labile'*; they may break into tears without provocation, or be euphoric. Some are irritable, or described as 'changed' by friends and family.

♦ *Depression occurs sometimes, but not often.* It differs from primary typical depression in that hedonia (loss of the sense of pleasure), anxiety and insomnia are uncommon. The depressive symptoms most closely resemble those seen in chronic, medical or neurological illnesses. Hypochondriasis is common; patients may bring long lists of symptoms to their clinic visits.

♦ A small minority of patients have *neurological signs* which are often short-lived and do not in any sense 'explain' the remainder of the syndrome.

CFS is usually readily recognizable. It is important to be aware of other types of physical illness in which fatigue is a major symptom, with which it can sometimes be confused. Michael Sharp, honorary consultant in psychological medicine at Edinburgh University, describes what these might be:

♦ If you have a lot of joint and muscle pain, your doctor may do tests for a range of rheumatic diseases. They are 'auto-immune' diseases (where the body's own immune system causes damage to bodily organs) and often cause joint pain and fatigue.

♦ Some gut disorders may lead to fatigue. These usually also cause diarrhoea and weight loss. If you have predominant gastric symptoms, your doctor may arrange for tests to exclude such conditions.

♦ Neurological diseases can present with fatigue. Multiple sclerosis usually causes loss of power or sensation in part of the body, while myasthenia gravis is a rare condition in which there is a problem between the muscles and the nerves that make them work. Both are treatable.

♦ Hormonal conditions can lead to fatigue. A routine test of urine/blood glucose for diabetes may be appropriate, as may a blood test for an underactive thyroid gland. An endocrine condition called Addison's disease (due to inadequate function of the adrenal gland) also causes fatigue, but is very rare. Giving the missing hormone can treat all these conditions.

♦ Infections can certainly cause fatigue. Examples include viral hepatitis, Lyme disease, glandular fever and Q fever.

♦ Severe sleep problems such as a condition called sleep apnoea syndrome can cause daytime fatigue, mainly sleepiness. Sleep apnoea is when a person stops breathing briefly many times during the night, which is often associated with loud snoring. It is diagnosed by having sleep and breathing measured overnight in a sleep laboratory and is treatable.

These medical conditions usually exhibit other symptoms which act as a clue to the underlying problem. There is, however, always a catch where fatigue is the *only* symptom of the underlying physical illness, and without other pointers as to what is going on the diagnosis may be overlooked for months or even years. This is illustrated by the following three examples.

Coeliac Disease

Coeliac disease is an inflammation of the lining of the gut, due to sensitivity to gluten in wheat and is usually associated with other appropriate bowel symptoms. Occasionally it may not be, as medical student Jo Bramall, described in the *British Medical Journal*:

> During my third year at medical school in Cardiff I gradually became unwell, with *depression, lethargy, exercise intolerance, muscle weakness, lack of motivation and a general lack of well*

being. When I finally consulted my family doctor I was told I was anaemic and should eat a proper balanced healthy diet. It was my flatmate, a registrar, who suggested that my diet may not be responsible. He suggested I was malabsorbing, might have Coeliac disease and should have my endomysial antibodies (specific tests for Coeliac disease) checked.

Eventually I got fed up with feeling ill and being nagged by my flatmate I went to my GP for the test which I learned a week later was positive. I was sent to a dietician and started on a gluten free diet. I am now unable to eat anything that contains wheat, rye, barley or oats. It surprised me how complicated that can be. I can eat potatoes, but not chips – they are contaminated with gluten from the batter on the fish fried in the same oil.

I feel so much better on this diet I can hardly believe how run down I was before. My energy levels have soared and I am now able to exercise regularly. Every time I am tempted by the look of a cake or the smell of freshly baked bread I just try to remember how I felt before my diagnosis.

Low Blood Pressure (Hypotension)

The recently described Postural Orthostatic Tachycardia Syndrome or POTS (low blood pressure associated with a fast heart rate) is a failure of the body's systems to respond to the increased demand on the heart posed by exercise. *Even mild exertion causes a raised heart rate, with an associated fall in blood pressure which is perceived as light headedness or weakness.* Not surprisingly this can be misdiagnosed as being due to CFS.

Hidden Infection

Mr N.M. from Torquay writes:

Early in 1996 my wife became very *lethargic and depressed*. Her doctor did all the usual tests which revealed nothing, but an acquaintance remarked that he had similar symptoms in the past which were traced to a septic tooth. My wife's dentist found an *abscess under an upper molar*. The tooth was removed and her lethargy rapidly cleared. It seems that because the trouble was in the upper jaw, there was no intense pain, so the infection was draining into her 'system'.

MUSCLE FATIGUE/WEAKNESS

Query 48-year-old Mrs E.N. from South Wales writes:

For the last five years I have had episodes of *weakness in my arms following (initially) hard work*. Only complete rest seemed to help. No numbness, no tingling, but plenty of odd sensations difficult to describe; heat sensation, a lesser sub-tingling feeling and an over-riding sensation of local exhaustion in the arms as though I had been hanging on for dear life to a branch. It is hard to relax the muscles, they keep tensing unbidden which I feel hinders the rest which is essential to any improvement.

There is a time delay. Too much effort one day will be 'paid for' over the next few days. The energy drains out rapidly, but returns very slowly and never fully. This year I noticed a pattern: as the light reduces from late August, so less and less effort tips me down the slippery slope to the near helplessness I have been in for three Christmases (0.5 out of 10 on a subjective scale of function). Last summer the best I achieved was 5 out of 10 and that was only if I was a 'good girl' and didn't lift or do anything much. A neurologist found nothing wrong and I have been ricocheting around various alternative therapies.

Comment There are a variety of fairly well-recognized muscle conditions such as myasthenia gravis where, as here, the main symptom is of ready fatiguability of individual muscles. None, however, really fits with this detailed description. The nearest is Pompe's disease, where the muscle is unable to use its store of glycogen and the only therapy is a diet utilizing another source of energy, protein.

Two readers comment:

- ♦ 'These symptoms resemble my son's problem, who has Pompe's disease. The only treatment is a high protein diet as exercise draws protein from the muscles and so stored glycogen cannot be retrieved for energy.'
- ♦ 'My arms have been affected in a similar fashion to Mrs E. I had to do very little to become fatigued and lose all muscle power. I spent days in bed. Despite all the usual neurological tests no diagnosis was forthcoming. I reluc-

tantly consulted an alternative practitioner who put me on daily protein supplements. I felt a positive reaction after a month and now six months later feel better than I have for the last five years.

Alternatively, another reader suggests that the problem is a failure to absorb vitamin B6.

I too have been investigated for mystery muscle weakness by many doctors and have been tested for myasthenia, MS, ME and potassium deficiency. All drew a blank. I consulted a nutritionist at a local complementary centre, who told me my body could not absorb vitamin B6 properly and advised me to take a supplement. My symptoms of weakness in all my muscles disappeared overnight. I was astounded to find a simple alternative to be the answer after eight years of poor health.'

Finally, there is some similarity between Mrs E.N.'s symptoms and the following case of a 35-year-old man with muscle pain on exertion, as described by Dr John Walton from Newcastle:

In his late 20s he had first experienced dull painful aching in the calf and thigh muscles, coming on after prolonged exertion and generally towards the end of the day. If he rested, the pain would disappear over a few hours and was invariably relieved by a night's sleep, however prolonged and intense the preceding exertion. Gradually, however, the muscle aching increased and spread after three years to his thighs, buttocks and hamstrings and then to his arms, hands and shoulder girdle. In time the pain became almost constant, with only slight relief resulting from rest. His sister, who is four years older, had had identical symptoms.

Investigations were normal and the patient's condition and that of his sister thus remained unexplained. He was started on the drug Verapamil 60mg three times a day. The response was immediate and dramatic, with remarkable relief of his muscle pain and tenderness within 26 hours – and his sister has been similarly helped.

MUSCLE PAIN/STIFFNESS

Query 78-year-old retired civil engineer Mr D.J. from Hampshire writes:

For some 20 years *I have had increasing muscular pain chiefly in my neck, head, arms, thighs and buttocks similar to the feeling of acute stiffness after, say, cross-country running, but painful without movement.* I get spasm in the upper centre of my back and in my abdomen. My wife, who has seen my back, says it is knotted. This has the result of my never being able to sit in a chair or lie in a bed comfortably. Periodically, despite a sleeping pill, I am forced to get up for a hour or so in the night and then again try to get to sleep. The evenings are the worst, though I have had it when I wake up, although it eases once I am up and moving about. Also I have had smarting eyes since about 18. Orthodox medicine from my sympathetic doctor and consultant cannot help further. Currently I take two Amitriptyline pills at night. I have also tried morphine with little or no success. Over the years I have tried faith healers, hynotherapy, homeopathy, vegetarianism, iridology, reflexology and chiropracters, at times cut out dairy products, gluten and my limited consumption of alcohol, but with no improvement.

Comment This is a most difficult problem for which there were few suggestions. It has some similarities to a condition known as the muscular pain-fasciculation syndrome. This is thought to be due to an inflammation of nerves, though here – as in the previous mystery – the symptoms tend to be brought on by exercise. Dr Arthur Hudson of the University of Western Ontaria describes them as follows:

The pain is usually present in more than one region, but most often in the legs, notably the calf. The pain varies in intensity from mild to severe. It was described as a constant ache, occasionally burning, and occurred following periods of physical activity or at the end of a working day. Fasciculation (muscle twitching) is first noticed about the same time as, or a year or two after, the onset of the pain. This is observed as solitary twitches of leg muscles, which move from place to place over larger areas of the body.

Further suggestions were as follows:

Underactive Thyroid

'I have very similar symptoms – violent spasms in the middle back which are quite painful, and aches all over the body, especially in the neck and shoulders, leading to total discomfort in bed. When I was diagnosed as having an underactive thyroid and given thyroid replacement therapy all this faded except for a tendency to sudden shivering.'

Polymyalgia

Dr Tony Betts from Watford writes:

> The possibility crossed my mind this may be due to polymyalgia rheumatica. Although all investigations have been negative, this condition can certainly occur before the age of 60 and may occasionally be associated with a normal ESR. The therapeutic test to prove diagnosis one way or another is a trial of oral Prednisolone. A moderate dose of 15–20mg will produce a distinctive improvement within 48 hours.

Food Intolerance

'My similar symptoms seems to be related to food intolerance. It started off with minor twinges, which I put down to 'getting older' – as one does. Then I realised I was having trouble getting out of the bath, going downstairs and other normal daily functions. I looked at my 80-year-old mother and realized she had none of my difficulties, so it wasn't old age. My wife suggested taking the so-called stone age diet and – eureka – that was it! After all the procrastination I tried it. Bingo. I hated it but that was the answer. In my case it appears to be yeast that causes the problem. This means not eating all the things I like best – cheese, fresh bread, beer and worse of all, no vino. So unfair. If I do cheat, it returns smartly. When I give up the poisoned chalice it takes a good week to regain the benefits, with definite withdrawal symptoms every time.'

Dystonia

'I wonder if your correspondent with the general muscle spasms has some form of dystonia. I have had this condition for nearly 20 years and have met many other sufferers whose symptoms are very diverse.'

Acupuncture

'Several years ago I found a very hard deep pressure from a pointed stick could give relief – but this also caused severe bruising and swelling – but I found it preferable to the muscle spasm. I have now found I can relieve the spasms reasonably effectively by using acupuncture – self-administered with an electro-acupuncture piece of equipment called acupoint.'

DIFFICULTY STANDING AND WALKING

Query 1 Mrs G.B. from Evesham writes:

> *My problem is a total inability to stand or walk for more than about 30 minutes. It is as if a tap has been switched off and all the blood goes from my head.* I have had heart and circulation tests. Apart from only lasting for three minutes on a treadmill because my energy had been expended walking to the hospital from the car park, everything was deemed to be normal. In every other respect I am extremely healthy and had I more stamina would have been a good sportswoman. As it is I have gone through life like a geriatric Cinderella and I would love to know why.

Query 2 Mrs P.D. from Norfolk writes: 'For the last 14 years *I have had episodes where quite suddenly I am unable to walk. I can only describe it as though my "power supply" is cut off.* I stumble, feel exhausted and have to be helped to the nearest chair and sleep for several hours. These episodes last for about three months, after which mobility returns to normal.'

Comment These two problems of difficulty with walking are quite different but are both strongly suggestive of some psychological element, where Mrs G.B.'s symptoms are similar to chronic fatigue syndrome, while those of Mrs P.D. of some anxiety depressive disorder. The following possibility, however, might be considered.

Postural Orthostatic Tachycardia Syndrome (POTS)

This condition is of a fast heart rate and consequent low blood pressure, which is induced by standing or walking.

♦ 'The symptoms sound like orthostatic intolerance, which can be tested for by standing quietly next to a wall and not fidgeting. Before 30 minutes is up most sufferers will feel nauseous, pale, headachey and probably be in distress.'

♦ 'I have similar symptoms (to Mrs E.N.) and finally after two years of endless medical opinions, I was diagnosed with POTS. This is a complex neurological condition which is only now being thorough researched.'

DIZZINESS ON EXERTION

Query Mr F.H., former architectural representative from Southport writes: 'For at least 25 years I have been plagued by *regular bouts of feeling quite ill* – although I know there is nothing wrong with me so I press on regardless. The *main symptom is one of feeling flushed as if I have a temperature* and I have noticed over the years it can be brought on my overdoing gardening or DIY.'

Comment This mystery raised several interesting possibilities.

Angina

'The description 'feeling quite ill' states the problem precisely, but no one seems to recognize it as a known symptom of angina until I had a bad attack with much chest pain shooting up into the neck. Before that I kept being asked if I felt giddy and the answer was 'not particularly'. Generally recovery was after an hour or two, but I could feel shaky for as much as 24 hours. Squatting whilst gardening, as opposed to kneeling or bending, produces the most severe reaction. I am at present being treated for angina and the problem has greatly lessened.'

Gastric Acid Reflux

'My symptoms have been worse each time after a bending session. They produced a sudden severe pain (and irregular heart beats probably caused by anxiety) in my chest making me suspect a heart attack and ending up in hospital. This happened several times and was eventually diagnosed as gastric reflux. I was put on Lansoprazole which alleviated it, but if I have to bend it has to be done with the knees instead of the back.'

Neck Pain

'It might be worth considering a neck problem. This is sometimes overlooked, as it was when I had similar symptoms. After reading how physiotherapy could possibly help in the situation, I consulted a physiotherapist who told me that treatment for my neck was necessary. Within 2–3 weeks I was much better.'

POTS (again)

The following description is strongly suggestive of POTS (as described above.)

I had assumed I was the only person in the world suffering from this syndrome which I call, perhaps not very originally, exertion sickness. Not surprisingly I came to assume the condition was totally unknown to medical science! The symptoms was a feeling of giddiness which will come on following over-exertion. I first encountered the malady in my early 40s when frolicking with my young son. The symptom was usually fairly mild, but was unpleasant because it could last several days. Sometimes it could make me feel quite ill. It was exhaustively investigated by my GP and consultant and at one point I had an angiogram, but all to no avail. My main defence lay in endeavouring not to exceed the threshold at which the condition could be triggered. This was very difficult because although not an athlete, I always enjoyed vigorous exercise and the symptoms would not be manifested until the exertion was over. The worst single instance I recall occurred after I had helped a neighbour to push his broken-down car from the road into his driveway. In the middle of the night following, I got out of bed to urinate as usual and found myself crashing drunkenly around the room when feeling my way to the loo.

Excess Caffeine

'I too have suffered from the problem of feeling ill after gardening or DIY. It always occurs at weekends when people have the time to carry out such tasks, and after reading an article I realised that this was probably due to the effects of excess caffeine lowering the blood sugar levels. Thus during the working week it was one cup of coffee with breakfast before setting out and a further mug of instant at about 11 o'clock at work which was fairly sedentary. At weekends, especially Sunday, there was time for a second mug of coffee and a further one before elevenses. Since I have confined myself to one mug at breakfast and taking some other beverages for elevenses I have not had a single reoccurrence. The bouts of feeling ill always coincided with some DIY or gardening which is very physical. Resting and taking some high sugar food usually corrected the problem after 40 minutes or so.'

TIREDNESS ON RISING

Query 1 Mrs F.M. from Chelsea writes:

It happens occasionally that I wake to an empty day feeling more than usually calm, energetic and full of ideas and plans for things to accomplish. *I start enthusiastically, but by nine or ten experience a collapse with head foggy, 'drained' feeling stomach and legs and my neck tight at the back, fit only to read.* This can last for the rest of the day. It has happened on and off over the past 50 years and results in a deplorably inhibited outlook.

Query 2 Mrs C.E. from Surrey writes: '*After a good night's rest I wake up feeling fine. About half an hour later an overwhelming fatigue sweeps over me and it needs all my willpower to shake myself up and ignore it.* On a few occasions when I have not succeeded in doing so I have woken up one hour later slumped over my crossed arms onto the breakfast table!'

Query 3 Mrs K.M. from Wrexham writes: 'Every morning when I get up I feel fine, but in about half an hour I am *overcome with extreme tiredness and my legs feel weak*. This can persist for some time but if I override it and force myself to do some gardening or go for a swim, very soon I feel OK again.'

Comment Most doctors confronted by this type of tiredness would almost certainly suspect that it was 'psychological' and prescribe antidepressants. Still, the similarity and specificity of the nature of the tiredness does point to some physical explanation. This could be a manifestation of some sleep disorder resulting in daytime tiredness caused by restless or burning legs, or when associated with snoring, the condition of obstructive sleep apnoea. Two further possibilities were suggested:

Carbon Monoxide Poisoning

'I would suggest that the lady might have any gas appliances checked over – water heater, fires and ovens – and also the ventilation, particularly in respect of the areas in which she spends the first half hour after rising.'

Aluminium Sensitivity

'I would suggest the problem is the gas given off by heated aluminium. It comes from heated saucepans, reflective or ornamental aluminium heaters and the sun on aluminium window frames or greenhouses. In big buildings the hot air may be ducted through aluminium pipes and may be a cause of sick building syndrome.'

16
Shivering, Hot and Cold Sweats

This section covers a wide spectrum of conditions involving raised temperature, perceptions of inner temperature – whether hot or cold – and unusual patterns of sweating.

WINTER (AND BATH-INDUCED) SHIVERS

Query 67-year-old retired bookseller Mr T.J. from Oxford writes:

> Here's an odd thing. In the winter months only, November to February, *four hours after I have had a bath I shiver uncontrollably no matter how many clothes I wear or how close to a fire I may be.* On getting into bed I run a temperature and have nightmarish dreams. The whole of the next day I am well below par. My family doctor says he hasn't come across this before and doesn't think it indicates anything serious. He may be right – but it's very unpleasant.

Comment The seasonality of these symptoms and association with bathing would suggest some problem with the mechanisms of temperature control – where cooling the body is followed by a compensatory rise in temperature. I was unable to identify any reports of this condition, but several readers report variations on the theme.

♦ Mrs C.J. from Wiltshire writes: 'I also suffer severe

uncontrollable shivering – but mine starts about three to four hours after visiting any of the local swimming pools for a session in the water. I used to attend twice a week for exercise and after three times I suffered the coldness and shivering and total incapacity necessitating going to bed and using extra blankets for warmth. This then started happening after every visit until "the penny dropped". I ceased to go swimming and since this time I have had no further occurrence.'

♦ Mrs J.B. from Leicester writes: 'My symptoms relate to falls in air temperature during December to February. If it is very cold outdoors I avoid going out if at all possible and if the house temperature falls, although I do not shiver I am unable to get warm. The cold seems to be inside my being. I need to warm up from the inside out.'

RECURRENT FLU

Mr A.G. from Sussex writes:

Three years ago *I had a severe attack of flu that appeared to recur three or four times over the next 12 months*. Subsequently it became progressively more frequent, as now at fortnightly intervals or less. Symptoms are virtually identical each time. I feel cold and shivery, then hot and weary, I start coughing and have a slightly sore throat. My nose drips and my bowel motions become more frequent. The nose drips cease, the cough becomes worse and my head feels very tight. After some hours – or a day or so – the head clears and for the time being I feel all right, but seldom lose the cough completely. In order to be certain of being fit enough to keep any engagement or holiday, this has to be fixed in advance.

Comment This certainly sounds like recurring bouts of flu, but again I was unable to find any descriptions of a similar syndrome. Two further readers report the same phenomenon.

♦ Mrs M.A. from Kent: 'I caught last winter's flu but my symptoms never completely "came out". Once a week for 12 weeks I had the same flu-like symptoms – shivering followed eventually by hot temperature, extreme fatigue – especially in the evening. This would last for a day or so then there would be a gap of three weeks and now three months before repeated bouts.'

♦ Mrs F.M. from Kent: 'I have been troubled with a virus for the past 16 years and have never come across anyone with the same problem. I was staying with my daughter and grandson when they both fell ill with a type of flu. I was also taken ill with a burning face which did not appear red and I felt extremely ill, with a temperature of 103°F. I had no aches or pains, no sweats and with the help of aspirin after about ten days I was able to return home. Subsequently I have had repeated returns of this trouble about twice a year for two to three years. Each time I have visited my grandson this burning face recurred and I was quite ill with a temperature. My doctor called it grandmother/grandson syndrome and I would gradually grow out of it. It has attacked me so often now, usually about every couple of years. I always get the burning face and quite a lot of nasal clear mucus and feel quite ill. It hangs around usually for three weeks and I take aspirin or paracetemol and lots of fluid.'

PYREXIA OF UNKNOWN ORIGIN (PUO)

A pyrexia of unknown origin is defined as an illness of at least three weeks' duration with fever (temperature exceeding 38.3°C on several occasions) and no established diagnosis, despite one week of hospital investigation. Its main feature is, of course, the temperature, without any suggestive hints in the form of other symptoms to identify its source. When the cause is eventually identified, it, not surprisingly, usually turns out to be some form of hidden infection or exotic illness (often acquired abroad) or some inflammatory disease like rheumatoid arthritis.

'Hidden' Bacterial Infection

There are many potential 'hiding places' for bacteria, including the gall bladder and the teeth.

♦ *Gall Bladder*

(i) '*My mother would start to shiver, become very cold and eventually go to bed with two or three hot water bottles. After a while she would begin to sweat and get very hot until the bed was more or less soaked.* This went on for about four hours then she cooled down, but was totally washed out the next day. Her symptoms completely mystified her doctor and she never had any pain. It wasn't until she was in hospital having a check-up for something else and had an attack there that somebody got the clue as to what the cause might be. She was found to have gall stones which were removed and she never had another attack.'

(ii) 'My father had short-lived episodes of high temperature and intense shivering without any associated pain. They proved difficult to diagnose, but eventually the symptoms were attributed to blockage of the bile duct and associated local infection. It required a major operation in which a highly infected gall bladder was removed. Thanks to the surgeon's skill he survived this very serious illness.'

♦ *The Teeth*

Dr Yecheskel Samra from Tel Aviv University describes the following case:

A 57-year-old man was admitted to hospital with a persistent fever of 38°C. Thorough investigation failed to identify a cause and because of the possibility of drug fever, all medications were discontinued – but the fever persisted. He had a therapeutic trial of the antibiotic Chloramphenicol which resulted in the patient's temperature returning to normal – but it promptly returned when the course was finished. After a month of investigation he began to complain of pain in his teeth. Examination revealed advanced peridontitis (inflammation of the tissue supporting the teeth). The teeth were extracted and the pyrexia resolved gradually. One year after discharge he remained symptom free.

Exotic Infections

There are numerous exotic infections that can be contracted while abroad or from animals with which doctors are usually unfamiliar, resulting in a delay in diagnosis. These include brucellosis, leptospiros, Q fever, Lyme disease and many others. A family doctor from the north west of England, who spent a month in Saudi Arabia, describes his experience with brucellosis. 'It was great – five-star luxury, trips to the desert and the skin diving in the Red Sea was divine.' A fortnight after his return, however, '*I developed rigors during the night. The chills came first, then I was cold, very cold and I covered myself with blankets. The shakes followed.* The morning found me caked in sweat.' His consultant ordered a 'complete batch of tests' and everyone sat back to await the results.

A week passed and the rigors continued, but no diagnosis was made. 'The consultant went off on holiday and I was left to the mercy of his registrar, who wanted to do a liver biopsy.' He managed to dissuade him from doing this and instead suggested that he might contact the hospital in Saudi Arabia to find out if anyone else had gone down with a similar mysterious illness. 'I was in my second week of hospitalization and had lost 22lbs in weight when the diagnosis finally arrived. Brucellosis was prevalent in Jeddah and I had attended the delivery of a Bedouin woman with a fever. The midwife, the nurse and myself had all caught brucellosis from her. A quick course of Tetracycline cured the rigors but it was six months before I regained my weight and previous state of health.' [Brucellosis is caused by the bacterium brucella melintensis which gains entry to the body through the tissues of the mouth and pharynx and spreads through the bloodstream to cause rigors and debility. Following the acute illness it can remain in the body to cause recurring symptoms over many years.]

Rheumatism and Other Inflammatory Conditions

Following the decline of infectious diseases over the last 50 years, accelerated by the double onslaught of better hygiene and antibiotics, the proportion of PUOs attributed to infections has fallen, and inflammatory conditions such as rheumatism are now much more frequently incriminated.

Query Retired Army chaplain the Reverend T.S. from North Wales writes:

> Throughout the whole of my career I thankfully enjoyed very good health and was very fit. I served mainly in the UK and on the Continent and from time to time I did tours of duty in Northern Ireland, Saudi Arabia and other countries. My symptoms are as follows. I experience *a day or two of complete weariness followed by aching limbs (slightly) which then feel very heavy*. This feeling culminates in the most *debilitating rigor* attack with extreme inner coldness and strong involuntary shivering. Such rigors can last for 15–40 minutes. Then there follows a period of *heavy sweating* which can remain with me for hours, often soaking thoroughly nightwear and bedding. Sometimes more than once per night. Many of these attacks are accompanied by a *lurid deep red rash* spreading across my buttocks or across the genital area. This is painless and does not itch.
>
> Nothing seems to allay this malady nor ease the awful ill feeling. Antibiotics, paracetemol, aspirin seem not to help and one must ride it out. The attacks can be of a 'one off' kind within a day or night, or come as a series (sometimes up to four) over a period of a few days. This leaves me feeling so ill and depressed, very weak and listless. I have often lost 5–8lbs in weight over a period of an attack. It can then take up to two weeks to return to normality.

Comment This unfortunate gentleman had every conceivable investigation during two separate admissions to the Liverpool School of Tropical Medicine. No diagnosis had been made. Two suggestions were put forward to explain these symptoms which had eluded the diagnostic skills of so many medical advisers. Both are inflammatory conditions and belong to the group known as connective tissue disorders or auto-immune disease, whose cause is not known but where the body's immune system is 'triggered' into attacking its own tissues.

♦ *Polyarteritis nodosa*: 'I would have either violent shivering attacks lasting 10–15 minutes followed by a similar period of "glowing" like an electric fire with my temperature over 100°. There then followed a period of profuse sweating which would soak clothing or sheets and blankets, which continued for 15 minutes when my temperature would return to normal, leaving me in a thoroughly washed-out condition. I also experienced a vivid red/purple rash on my lower trunk – the genitals and upper parts of my thigh. I spent some time in Northwick Park Hospital. After three or four weeks in an isolation ward the cause of my illness was recognized as being polyarteritis nodosa. I was given steroid tablets, which halted my downward path and set me on the road to recovery.'

♦ *Palindromic rheumatism*: 'My malarial-like attacks occur with frightening rapidity usually building up over a couple of minutes day or night. They last 40–45 minutes, never less, never more. The inner core of one's body seems to turn to ice, although the outer temperature seems to remain normal. No matter what clothing you add or however you try to warm up – nothing works. As suddenly as it starts it declines, until you just slump exhausted. The intense shivering and shaking leaves you drained. There is then 15–20 minutes of calm until the sweating begins. It is not uncommon for a change of pyjamas and bedding twice in a night – sometimes several nights in a row. I already suffer from arthritis and the pain in my shoulders and knees now became severe. The attacks occurred every six weeks or so and lasted about a week. The pain in the shoulder and knees gradually tapering down to a steady ache at the end. The family doctor sent me to a consultant rheumatologist who gave me a thorough examination, listened carefully to my tale of woe and without any hestitation diagnosed palindromic (episodic) rheumatoid arthritis and prescribed Hydroxychloroquine tablets, two per day. This drug is not a miracle cure but has gradually brought my problem under control.'

There are, not surprisingly, numerous other possible sources of a PUO including hidden cancers of the colon, bladder, oesophagus or ovary, drug side effects, other inflammatory conditions and the unusual genetic condition of Familial Mediterranean Fever.

TOTAL BODY SWEATS

Query 1 80-year-old farmer's wife, Mrs W.B. from Taunton writes: 'I suffer *continual sweats* which seem to get worse as I grow older. They occur, for no apparent reason, over a dozen times a day. My doctor can suggest no cause nor anything to alleviate them.'

Query 2 Mr T.V. from Pinner writes:

> I too experience these sweats which are definitely *not* like menopausal flushes. As you can imagine hot weather is complete torture for us. As far as I am concerned, it is windows and curtains closed and stay in the house all day. Also, I am never cold. I am the only one to be walking about in the winter with no coat and almost everywhere is too hot for me. My first consideration when I am going anywhere is what can I wear that will be cool enough. It is very unpleasant, not helped by the knowledge my mother suffered these sweats until she died recently at the age of 98.

Query 3 66-year-old Mrs M.R. from Hampshire writes: 'When I wake up and start to move about the first sweat arrives and they continue on and off throughout the day, and often makes sleep difficult. I feel I need to be in a continual breeze to live a comfortable life. Attending church is embarrassing as I literally drip – I have given up the theatre and concerts unless I can sit where there is a draught. Recently I have been getting palpitations during the night accompanied by the sweats.'

Query 4 59-year-old Mr H.C. from Malvern writes:

> These continual sweats have blighted my personal and professional life since my late 30s. I too have sadly given up church, concerts and theatres and when forced to attend, only feel really at

ease in the back row and in a draught. I too dread dinner parties and though I am not a total loner or unsociable I often find it convenient to give the impression I am so in order to avoid being invited. It was death to my chosen high-profile profession when I found myself avoiding meetings and formal entertaining. To an extent I too believe it might be inherited. I recollect my father often mopping his brow at such events as speech days and my mother dreaded even the simplest social occasion, saying that she got 'so hot' – though she did not break into sweats. As a child I used to blush very easily, but not sweat abnormally. For long now I have sweated unusually heavily with the mildest physical exertions such as walking or working in the garden. I am seldom cold, even in winter.

Comment The source of these very distressing total body sweats are not well understood – though they can be a feature of the readily diagnosed condition of an overactive thyroid or thyrotoxicosis. They point to a disturbance in several different ways of the temperature regulating (thermoregulatory) mechanisms to the body. The female sex hormones play a role – hence the hot flushes and heavy sweating that is so characteristic of the menopause. There may be a genetic element, as the condition seems to run in families. Further, there is obviously a degree of heat intolerance as suggested by the way the symptoms are exacerbated by hot weather and the observation that the sufferers 'never feel the cold'. There may also be a disturbance of the nervous control of the sweat glands and blood vessels of the skin to cause the flushing and heavy sweating. This is a more generalized phenomenon than the localized heavy sweating related to the armpits and hands, which is known as hyperhydrosis.

The general view is that the treatment options for whole body sweating are quite limited, but the following possibilities might be considered.

Hormonal

Several readers emphasise how these sweats are quite distinct from those experienced during the menopause, indeed they must be because of the way it can also affect men. Nonetheless, in some at least hormones must be implicated, as shown by the following observations:

- ◆ 'I too suffered from continual sweats for some time, until my doctor as a last resort suggested my going on to HRT by way of patches. This caused great hilarity to my family as I am 80 years old – however, it stopped the sweats!'
- ◆ 'I had hot flushes and night sweats when I was about 52 as I finished menstruating. I went on to HRT and the flushes stopped within a fortnight, so I continued for 12 years with no side-effects at all. I stopped last month to see what would happen and the flushes have started again. It therefore would seem that they have only been delayed.'

Diabetes

Heavy sweating is reported by one reader as an early symptom of diabetes:

I am 78 and three to four years ago I began to suffer sweats. The perspiration would be pouring off me – then it would go away only to start again after half an hour or so. Some time after they started I was found to be suffering from non-insulin dependent diabetes. I was given a diet sheet and testing strips but the sweating didn't really go away until I was put on glicazide. Now it still happens but not nearly so badly.

Drug Side-Effects

It is conceivable that excess sweating may be a side-effect of the beta blockers readily prescribed for angina and raised blood pressure: 'The same problem started immediately after a heart attack three years ago, when I was prescribed the beta blocker Atenolol by the hospital. I progressively cut the dosage in an attempt to circumvent the sweating and then I still sweated quite badly. It is certainly much improved.'

Autonomic Nervous System

The autonomic nerves control the production of sweat by the sweat glands and the calibre of the blood vessels in the skin. The neurotransmitter acetylcholine is involved, and it is possible that some relief can be obtained by blocking its action.

(i) *Belladonna* 'I mentioned night sweats to my osteopath who said "I can cure that" and gave me little Belladonna pills, one a day for ten days, then one if I had a sweat. Miraculous! Previously I would sit at breakfast or at the bridge table with my face dripping. Very embarrassing. Very rarely do I get them now – and if I do, one pill does the trick!'

(ii) *Antidepressants*: Certain antidepressants such as Amitriptyline also block the action of acetylcholine, producing the side-effects of dry mouth and reducing sweating.

Sage

'By accident I found a remedy for my nocturnal upper body perspirations that have plagued me for the past three years. It is the herb drink Bioforce Menosan whose active ingredient is sage. It should be taken as 15 drops in water once a day at teatime.'

FACIAL SWEATS AND FLUSHES

There are four distinct types of facial sweats, each of which illustrates one or other of the mechanisms already described.

Facial/Head Perspiration

Query 1 70-year-old Mrs S.J. from Dorset writes: 'My sweats are confined to my head and face. *My hair becomes quite wet and sweat runs down my face in rivulets.* This very tiresome condition is becoming more frequent. It can start out of the blue, but physical exertion makes it much worse.'

Query 2 60-year-old Mrs B.B. from South London writes: 'My sweats seem to affect my head more than anywhere else.

Perspiration literally drips off my chin and onto the inside of my glasses, and if I comb my hair I look as if I have just been swimming. It can be extremely embarrassing and it is not confined to hot weather – although it is worse then.'

Query 3 65-year-old Mrs B.S. from Sussex writes: 'I am very active but whenever I get hot gardening or even ironing, my neck pours with sweat around the hairline. It is extremely inconvenient and also ruins my hairdo.'

Query 4 Mrs R.G. from Oxford writes: 'I have had severe sweating fits, to the point where it literally runs down my face and drops off my jaw. I really dread being asked to formal dinners, parties, etc. as to be observed mopping face or neck with a large handkerchief is not very glamorous.'

Comment This problem seems to lie somewhere between the total body sweats of the previous section and the condition of primary (i.e. cause unknown) hyperhydrosis (excess sweating), which is limited to one part of the body. The cause again is excess activity of the nerves that control the sweat glands. Once again, the treatment options are limited.

(i) *Sweatbands*: 'I perspire from the hairline towards my forehead. The sweat simply pours down onto my glasses and drips onto the ground. A few years ago I bought a towelling headband such as worn by tennis players and this has solved the problem entirely. As the band goes right round the head under the hair it should prevent the sweat from running down the neck.'

(ii) *Topical Glycopyrrolate*: Glycopyrrolate is a drug that blocks the action of the neurotransmitter acetylcholine which controls the action of the sweat glands. Dr D.C. Seukeran, dermatologist at Leeds General Infirmary, describes the effect of treatment on a 24-year-old man with a five-year history of excess sweating of the scalp and forehead.

The excess sweating severely limited his social activities and led to the loss of his job as a barman. He had already applied aluminium chloride (anhydrol) to his forehead but this had only partially helped, as the sweating had resumed within 20 minutes. An aqueous solution of glycopyrrolate was then tried on both scalp and forehead, and this led to a dramatic improvement, with complete control of the hyperhydrosis. Initially the patient applied this twice daily but found that once a day application worked just as well.

(iii) *Antidepressants*: These drugs, as discussed above, block the action of acetylecholine and so theoretically might be useful in this situation, though I have been unable to find any reports of its use.

Taste-Induced (Gustatory) Sweating

Query Mrs L.C. from Essex writes:

> My main trouble is that over the last few months *whenever I come into contact with an atmosphere where food has been fried I immediately start to sweat profusely but only on the face and scalp*. Initially this would only last for about 20 minutes and wasn't too bad, however it has worsened to the extent where the sweating can last for several hours following exposure. During this time I also feel cold and shivery, and although my face and scalp are very warm, bright red and sweating, the rest of my body, particularly my hands and feet, are cold to the touch. I do not have to eat the fried food for the sweating to come on, but either be in the atmosphere where frying is taking place or more recently just opening a packet of crisps has started the sweating off. I discovered that taking an antihistamine such as Clarytine will reduce the severity and duration of the symptoms – so wonder if this could be some form of allergy.

Comment The phenomenon of taste- (or smell-) induced sweating was first described in 1923 by the neurologist Lucie Frey, and indeed is sometimes known as Frey's syndrome. It is due to 'inappropriate' nervous connections to the sweat glands, which most often follows surgery to the parotid gland, but may occur out of the blue. Treatment is on similar lines as for flushing and sweating as mentioned in the previous section.

(i) *Glycopyrrolate*: Dr H.R. Steghuis from New Zealand describes the case of a 45-year-old woman who developed sweating on the left side of her face whenever she ate – causing 'significant social embarrassment'. When the problem first occurred her surgeon told her nothing could be done. In fact a number of treatments are available, including commercial anti-perspirants, aluminium chloride in alcohol and nerve block. None of these treatments are as simple and generally effective as topical glycopyrrolate. The patient commenced treatment with 1% formulations and these controlled her symptoms for up to five days, with the only adverse effect being an occasional dry throat.

(ii) *Amitriptyline*: Dr D.J. Eedy from Belfast describes the case of a 42-year-old woman with a five-year history of profuse facial sweating precipitated by perfumed smells.

A few minutes after smelling perfume, beads of sweat were observed, more profuse on the left side. Flushing or other abnormality of the skin was noted and the profuse excess sweating continued for some 30 minutes. She commenced on Amitriptyline 75mg daily and within a few days reported clinical improvement and sweating could not be elicited by asking the patient to smell strong perfume. The dose was subsequently reduced to 25mg daily and after three years she remained symptom free.'

(iii) *Botulinum toxin*: Botulinum toxin is a potent poison that when injected locally paralyses the action of individual nerves and is therefore increasingly used for conditions associated with nervous overactivity. Dr Abigail Arad-Cohen of the Voice and Swallowing Disorders Centre in New York reports its use in six patients, the only adverse effect being a 'temporary slight weakness of the upper lip' in one.

Facial Sweating and Flushing Confined to One Side

Professor James Lance, biologist from Sydney, Australia, describes the following case.

A 29-year-old male landscape gardener had always sweated and flushed on both sides of his face until two years previously, when his wife noticed the right side of his forehead and upper face was a bright red colour after a game of squash, while the left side appeared pale. This asymmetry persisted for about 20 minutes. Since that time, he flushed easily on exertion or sometimes at rest on a hot day with the flush involving chiefly the right side of the forehead, fading in intensity over the right side of the nose and the right cheek. At the same time the right side of the face, particularly the forehead, sweated more than the left whereas sweating remained symmetrical over the remainder of his body.

Professor Lance describes this phenomenon as one of the 'most mysterious and dramatic of the neurological syndromes', which for obvious reasons he has dubbed the Harlequin syndrome. This is due to a localized disturbance of the autonomic nerves that control the sweat glands and blood vessels in the skin.

Social Facial Flushing and Sweats

Query 1 Mrs K.J. from Cheshire writes: 'For some years I have suffered from what can only be described as *"hot flushes" – not menopausal – which affect my face only. They occur often on social occasions and I go very red in the face and my cheeks pour with perspiration*. I feel my head could literally explode and often I have a slight headache too. It has got so bad it now threatens to ruin my social life.'

Query 2 Mrs D.J. from North London writes: 'My face becomes very hot and red with a burning sensation and results in broken capillaries in my cheeks. Other than hot surroundings and the sun, I am unable to establish what brings it on. I have consulted many doctors. It looks a bit like rosacea, but is not.'

Query 3 Mrs B.I. from Richmond writes: 'I am an active 70-year-old and although I normally have a pale, dry skin, in hot weather my face burns bright red and the heat causes me great distress and embarrassment. I try to avoid going out during the hottest part of the day but this is not always possible.'

Comment This is an exaggerated manifestation of the common phenomenon of blushing when embarrassed or the centre of attention. It can also be induced by excess sun exposure, heat or other factors that cause facial flushing, such as hot foods, alcohol, the menopause and medication. Some unfortunate people are chronic blushers, in whom the slightest stimulus can crimson the face and often the front of the chest as well. In its extreme form, this can lead to erythrophobia – a painful fear of blushing – for which the only escape is to become a social recluse. The social anxiety associated with this fear of blushing is itself an exacerbating factor. So paradoxically one of the treatments for those with erythrophobia is to encourage them to try to blush as often as possible so they become desensitized and the number of serious blushing episodes should diminish. Herbal and conventional medicines, relaxation and cognitive therapy may help – but recently another option has become available, as described by Christer Drott, associated professor of surgery at the University of Gothenberg in Sweden. This involves a keyhole surgery where the nerve to the small blood vessels of the face is cut. The operation was originally pioneered for the treatment of profuse hand sweating, but was also reported to have the unexpected benefit of dramatically reducing blushing.

The procedure involves making a small incision in the armpit and severing the sympathetic nerve as it passes over the second and third rib. The procedure is then repeated on the other side. 'The best effect is achieved with rapid attacks of blushing. Gradual blushing or flushing is poorly controlled by this procedure,' Professor Drott observes.

BODY HEAT

Query 1 Mrs O.S. writing on behalf of her 78-year-old retired printer husband, writes:

Ever since my husband's heart valve operation he has suffered from a peculiar thing *where he feels boiling hot from the chest upwards and very cold from the chest downwards.* His temperature is normal but when I am close to him the heat from his upper part is as if I am standing near a fire. He feels as if his head will explode and it makes him feel so ill. He has been in hospital twice for three-day stints, but they can't find any reason for it and they say there is nothing they can do.'

Query 2 Mrs F.M. from Southampton writes: 'My husband had a large part of his large bowel removed 20 years ago, after which he developed a non-sweaty body heat – recently we have had to take to separate beds. I always know when it is raised by standing near him and feeling the heat and noticing his increased respiration.'

Query 3 Mrs S.A. from Dorset writes: 'I get a feeling of intense heat (not perspiration) over my upper body when I lie down in bed. I am perfectly normal when up and about. This has persisted over many years and is not due to the menopause. I cannot sleep under a duvet and have only two blankets and only a small amount of heat in the bedroom. Apart from this I am in good health.'

Query 4 Mrs F.J. from Nottinghamshire writes:

> During the past two years I have become very hot in bed, sometimes almost burning. I have barely any covers on and I do not perspire and my skin does not feel hot to the touch. I am long past menopause. During the night and when I wake up in the morning the tips of my toes and toenails hurt – but this wears off after getting up. At night I have very slight vibration in various parts of my body – mostly my arms and legs. I have been seen in hospital and told that this is an 'essential' tremor.

Comment There is no explanation for this distressing sensation, which has some similarity to burning legs syndrome. Again it would seem that the nerves involved in heat control must somehow be involved, but in one instance the explanation was more straightforward:

> For six years following a coronary bypass operation I experienced boiling sensations and hot flushes from my chest upwards – and

despite many tests and visits to my cardiologist, nothing untoward was detected. But then an angry lump appeared on the surface in the middle of my chest. This turned out to be a deep-seated abscess of the sternum, where the titanium wire stitches had been used to close it following my operation six years previously. The abscess and the wires were finally removed and I am happy to say I no longer experience any hot flushes or burning sensations. My whole well-being has improved immeasurably.

BODY CHILLS

Query 1 Mrs M.B. from East Sussex writes on behalf of her partner:

Now aged 80 my partner (male) suffered a minor stroke three years ago. His 'attacks' give no warning and can happen at any time of day and indeed on some occasions have woken him at night. In duration they last only for about ten to 30 seconds, some being much more severe than others, but are extremely unpleasant and quite frightening. *He complains his whole body (including the face) feels ice cold – he shivers and shakes all over.* He describes a feeling of his body gradually 'thawing out'. He also (for a few seconds) feels very nauseous. Once the attack passes he quickly recovers and feels fine. Some days he may have anything from one to four or five attacks.

Query 2 Mrs P.A. from Devon writes:

My chills – as I now call them – started one Sunday afternoon. *I feel I am chilled inside and out* and the only way I can cope on an immediate basis is to sit by the fire wrapped in a blanket and with a hot water bottle. This takes the edge off it. Sleep can be disturbed by chilling and the following day 99 per cent has gone to be replaced by sensitive skin and shaking inside and out. I feel generally debilitated, but after a good night's sleep at the end of day 2 life returns to much more as usual.'

Comment There were, regrettably, no responses to these two mystery syndromes beyond a letter reporting an experience similar to that of Mrs M.B.'s partner.

COLD LEGS – AND MIDRIFF

Query 1 Mrs M.P. from Canterbury writes on behalf of her husband: 'After sitting for any length of time, for example *watching television in the evening, his lower legs and feet are icy cold*. These usually warm up once he is lying down in bed.'

Query 2 Mrs P.M. from Cheltenham writes: 'I suffer from cold feet for most of the day even though I exercise by walking daily. My feet are only usually warm when I warm my shoes or slippers on the radiator or go to bed warming them with an electric blanket and bedsocks before removing both sources of heat. During the night and on waking my feet will be very warm.'

Query 3 Mrs N.M. from Cheshire writes: 'Whenever I am in a sitting position I have a feeling of intense cold in the region of my midriff (back and front). I do not experience this condition when standing or lying in bed. I have consulted three doctors with no diagnosis or advice.'

Comment Cold legs are usually perceived as being due to 'poor circulation' either from narrowing of the arteries to the legs or in association with Raynaud's phenomenon, where the hands go blue and icy cold with temperature. The problem here, however, would seem to be heightened sensitivity to the cold as the following comment suggest:

♦ 'From my experience during winter evenings in an open-plan house in Michigan and during frosty evenings in a pre-war house in Sussex, this problem is due to the much lower air temperature at floor level than at, say, knee height and above, whatever type of central heating one has. The feet and calves will soon chill when settling down to watch TV.'

♦ 'I suffered the same symptoms at the age of 72, with my circulation and every other imaginable problem of "old age". However, placing a thermometer at ankle level quickly solved the problem. I was sitting in a direct line of a "door to window" draught line which, at 12°C, was considerably lower than the ambient temperature of the room.'

This proposal, however, would not explain Mrs N.M.'s complaint of a cold torso, and chiropracter Bernard Masters suggests an alternative explanation, of pressure on the autonomic nerves as they come out of the spine: 'The fact that the gentleman has to lie down to improve the warmth of his lower legs would indicate a need to reduce the loading on his spinal column.'

COLD SWEATS

Query 87-year-old Mrs B.R. from Cheshire writes:

I developed a mystery affliction, *perspiring when it is cold. The back of my neck and upper half of my back feel tacky with perspiration* – though my clothes aren't wet with it. It makes me feel thoroughly off-colour, off my food and lacking in energy. My doctor could find nothing untoward. The condition continued to the end of April then subsided with the milder weather. But back it came at the end of September and I am still plagued with it.'

Comment This phenomenon of cold-induced profuse sweating was described back in the 1970s in two sisters whose grandfather had the same problem – thus suggesting there must be a genetic component, though this does not seem to apply in this lady's case. Dr E. Sohar from Tel Aviv University reports:

In normal people thermal sweating occurs at rest only at external temperatures above 24°C. At 18°C there is virtually no sweating but these sisters sweated profusely from the chest and back when exposed to cold temperatures (18°–12°) whereas other areas remained dry and reacted normally to warm and cold stimuli. There was some improvement with the drug Atropin, which blocks the action of the neurotransmitter acetylecholine.

17
Sleep

Sleep hath its own world
And a wide realm of wild reality
And dreams in their development have breath
And tears, and tortures and the touch of Joy.
                    Lord Byron: 'The Dream'

'Sleep hath its own world', and despite much scientific scrutiny, the causes and mechanism of this altered state of consciousness in which we pass a third of our lives remains deeply enigmatic. Not surprisingly then, the sleep state is associated with several mystery syndromes, some of which – burning feet, periodic leg movements, stabbing eye and rectal pain, throbbing nostril, pounding heart – feature elsewhere. Further, as pointed out in the Introduction, the identification of one sleep condition in particular – OSA or obstructive sleep apnoea, where obstruction of the airways (signalled by snoring) causes intermittent cessation of breathing (apnoea) at night, leading to daytime sleepiness – illustrates the central theme of this book: how clarification of unusual symptoms is an absolute requirement for their correct treatment. And here are a few more.

VIVID DREAMS AND VIOLENT SPASMS

Query 1 Mrs M.A. from Milton Keynes writes:

My husband, aged 65 *suffers from nocturnal spasms. He has always been restless at night but approximately a year ago he got very violent and actually hurt and bruised* me, which came to a head when I woke up on the floor! My husband is very strong for his age, still doing some physical farm work. He does not wake up or know that he is doing this unless I wake him and then he recalls dreams which usually entail chasing various animals or playing badminton.

Query 2 Mrs F.M. from West Yorkshire writes:

My father (1903–1971) was a very nice man leading an outdoor life which was totally normal. As long as I can remember, his physically and mentally violent dreams were quite a joke in the family except to my mother trying to sleep with him. They usually had twin beds. A typical scenario he recounted was that he was on a railway engine which was travelling at speed and he was climbing all over the outside trying to get away from a Chinaman who was pursuing him with an axe. The dream would, of course, manifest itself in huge jerks and kicks, mainly with legs, because I do not remember he ever punched my mother.

Comment There is an obvious similarity between these descriptions and those of jumping legs (periodic leg movements), though the twin distinguishing features are the associated violent dreams and the 'total body' nature of the spasms. There are two possible diagnoses:

Rapid Eye Movement (REM) Sleep-Behaviour Disorder

Rapid Eye Movement here refers to the stage of sleep associated with dreaming, when the eyes move very rapidly from side to side. Dr Carlos Schenck of the Sleep Disorder Centre at the University of Minnesota describes a typical case:

A 57-year-old salesman had a normal quiet nocturnal sleep pattern for 52 years, when he began to talk, yell, move his limbs and sit up during sleep. After two years he also began to punch, kick and jump out of bed with progressive frequency and intensity. These behaviours, which always occurred at least two hours after sleep onset, were often attempted enactments of dreams which had become more vivid, action filled and antagonistic: 'Usually something is scaring me or is going to hurt my family and I try to protect them, then I get the most violent'. He had repeatedly struck and bruised his wife's arms and back and once punched through a wall while dreaming. During business trips he was continually embarrassed by the nocturnal activity.

Dr Antonio Culebras of the New York College of Medicine elaborates:

RSBD is characterized by a history of bizarre acts during nocturnal sleep ranging from muscle twitches, jerks and restlessness to complex forms of organized motor activity, such as flailing of arms, pointing with a finger, waving with a hand, punching, kicking, vocalizing, sitting up or getting out of bed, walking, running, screaming and jumping. This activity can lead to physical injuries to the patient or spouse. If awakened they report having a dream that drove them to act in their sleep. The character is usually violent featuring persecution and confrontation with persons or animals. Repetitive themes are common. It has been suggested these are quasi-intentional motor activities that might be an attempt to enact the dream content, which is frequently violent, vivid and confrontational. The treatment is with the drug Clonazepam which is highly effective in almost 90 per cent of cases.'

Parkinson's Disease

Similar nocturnal bizarre acts can occur as a feature of Parkinson's disease.

♦ 'Over the last three years or so my partner would shake and twitch violently several times a night and occasionally would kick or hit me. The episodes were often associated with violent dreams in which he would be having a fight or kicking something. Often he would shout out quite clearly in his sleep. Of course when he did this I woke him. I always got as far away as possible when he started trembling, knowing I might get hit or kicked. A few weeks ago he was diagnosed as having Parkinson's disease and the second night after starting treatment was marked by complete absence of the movement. I am pleased to say that since then my nights have been much more peaceful.'

♦ 'I am 79 and have had a tremor in my left hand for perhaps 20 years which has been diagnosed as Parkinson's disease. Privately over the last few months my wife tells me that sometimes I twitch and jerk during the night. Often I am unaware of this but sometimes recall dreaming. On occasions I have 'terror' dreams such as being attacked by, for example, wild animals, resulting in my lashing out. Since these seem to occur when I am sleeping on my left side my wife is in the line of fire.'

♦ 'My husband was diagnosed with Parkinson's two years ago and for about five years before that had been experiencing violent dreams (with spasms) to the extent he would be saving a goal for England and my head would be the rugby ball, or he would be trying to save me from baddies in dark glasses and raincoats, but I would be the one being bashed up. It would take me all my strength to restrain him.'

There is a further, more severe variation of this syndrome, reported by two readers, where the violent movements occur both at night and during the day and for which, despite intensive investigations, neurologists have been unable to make a specific diagnosis.

♦ Mrs J.C. from Ruislip writes: My hands or legs would shake violently, moving so fast that if I had been a boy scout I could have made fire. At night conscious convulsions and spasm would rip across my body five or six times a night, often throwing me across the bed. Spasms lock the hands and arms tightly across the body. Twice I was admitted to A&E and an MRI scan of head and neck was done. I spent three days in Charing Cross Hospital with an EEG linked to a video camera continuously day and night. Ten months on it is still in the body but not so severe or frequent. It is now a major problem in the head and face. The head shakes violently and the muscles in the face contort and the throat is also affected. It has baffled top neurologists and they are hoping if they look the other way it will pass from my body. But will it?

♦ Mr H.W. from Stockport writes: I am 73 years of age. Fifteen years ago I fell into a cellar opening being caught by my shoulders, which resulted in my spine 'springing'. There was damage to the nerves with a feeling of fire running up and down the spine. It was more than two years before I found a neurologist who knew what it was about and I had emergency surgery with a decompression operation. I was told I had been within a week of total paralysis from the neck down. Since then I have developed a permanent shake in my hands and arms and have suffered badly with spasm throwing me out of bed; locking my arms across my chest; throwing me forwards and sideways. The treatment for a spasm is for a family member to force me into an upright position; force my arms apart and force my hands open as if holding an object, and flex my spine in the opposite direction and hold me there until the spasms have passed, which they do up to a minute later.

I admit to surprise at the ignorance of my condition by members of the medical world. Doctors have run out of examination rooms when I have gone into spasm and said how frightened they were. The same applies to my lawyers when I suffered a spasm in their presence. My home has been altered and extended to allow me to live downstairs and avoid the use of stairs as my feet sometimes stick as I am walking upstairs.

VIGOROUS NOCTURNAL SENSORY SPASM

Query 72-year-old retired radiographer Mrs D.J. from Hertforshire writes:

For the last ten years I have had the following symptoms, which always happen in bed – the occurrence is intermittent but if spread over a year it never gets less nor more frequent, possibly six times. *It starts as a tingling beginning in my feet, slowly intensifying it works its way up to my head, where it 'blasts off' with a whirling dizziness.* It is something like an orgasm but considerably more violent. I am then perfectly normal again. It feels as though I jump in the bed but suspect I do not. Occasionally I have had the whole episode for a second time but that is very rare. It always happens after I have been drinking red wine but is not associated necessarily with every time I have red wine.

Comment This must rank as one of the most curious of all the mystery syndromes and may be a variation of the visual and sensory 'hypnagogic' hallucinations that may occur at the onset of sleep. Another reader describes it as being like an 'electric shock – a quick jab of my heart then going through my body. It was all over in seconds'. Nonetheless there were three further accounts of what is almost certainly the same syndrome that occurred while awake.

♦ Mrs M.R. from Devon writes: 'I had a similar experience in the reverse direction in the days following a hysterectomy operation at the age of 47. Here the tingling started not in the feet but at the tip of my scalp, progressed down my body, pushing out my arms to fingertips, down to my operation scar. The first time this happened I thought the stretching (which I was powerless to stop) would burst the scar open! There was absolutely no pain and the force continued down my legs, so that I had to stretch them and my toes, from whence it disappeared, leaving me exceedingly relaxed but wondering what it was. This happened perhaps two or three times a day for a week or so and gradually disappeared after about four weeks. I asked my yoga teacher what she thought it might be and her answer was I had indeed been very lucky to experience this and thought it was a shakra, an energy force helping me to get well.'

♦ 'I too have a sensation in my abdomen/chest/arms which I can only liken to an explosion of hot tingles like the popping of a champagne bottle. The sensation of hot bubbles then tingles through my chest and down both arms and frequently up my neck towards my face. This lasts for about a minute. These episodes occur in bed when I have been curled up in one position for some time and upon changing position the "hot explosion" occurs. It also happens if I have been slumped in an easy chair for any length of time and when I change position I get the same sensation.'

♦ Mr B.A. from Salisbury writes: 'Many years ago after a motorcycle tour of France I began to be troubled by a very insistent itch on my inside left ankle, which affected an area the size of a one penny piece. Although I was very good at keeping my fingers off the patch it grew about twice the size. If I succumbed to the insistence and scratched it quickly developed into a physical climax that surged right up to my head and face and was much more intense than a sexual climax. This was immediately followed by a most intense pain which slowly dissipated. The pain was quite sufficient to counter any notion of using the scratching to bring about the climax effect. When the dermatologist eventually treated the itchy patch it disappeared, never to return.

Comment The cause of these phenomena is of course quite obscure, though Mrs D.J. clearly associates it with drinking red wine and another reader linked it to liquorice. The concept of an 'energy force' as described by Mrs M.R. is elaborated by another reader.

This sensation is one which many would envy. It is the rising energy up the spine of the Kundalini serpent, a practice long known and understood from ancient times in India. Many mystics go into deep meditation to encourage this experience. It can, however, occasionally become very violent and cause both physical and mental distress. I experienced a 'triple rising' some years ago without knowing what it was and thought I must have had some kind of fit. Although a very practical salesperson and totally non-religious, I was somehow propelled into a spiritual healing. Please believe me, I am not a New Age nut. I am a 70-year-old grandmother of the old school and literally my life stopped.

Dr Jean Galbraith of St Albans elaborates:

I would suggest this is almost certainly a small regular spontaneous Kundalini rising experience up the spine. Some people suffer more acute and dramatic Kundalini rising events, a significant proportion of whom are sent to psychiatric hospitals with mania, psychosis and depression. This is a pathway suffered by saints such as St Theresa. The phenomenon was studied by Karl Jung with great interest. One result of such episodes is that the sufferer may acquire one or more spiritual gifts, e.g. healing, clairvoyance or literary gifts.

'HORRIBLE' SENSATION ON WAKING

Query 1 85-year-old housewife and gardener Mrs B.M. from Surrey writes:

Six years ago I started getting the most horrible sensation going through my body every time I woke from sleep, be it 4.00 a.m. or after a five-minute kip after lunch. It is difficult to describe but *is rather like poisoned soda water bubbles in the bloodstream* and sometimes the waking is traumatic, especially when in a chair or on the beach. In the daytime the effects work off more quickly if I mow the lawn.

Query 2 Mrs M.J. from York writes:

For varying periods of time – a few days to a few weeks – I am awakened from sleep in the early morning by a *very unpleasant sensation which flows through me*. It may only last a minute or so but may be repeated several times over my remaining time in bed. It seems to emanate from the area of my stomach/abdomen, spreading throughout my body, and can best be described as the sort of feeling one gets when receiving a shock, but it is intensely unpleasant – frightening in fact – and phrases like 'my heart jumped into my mouth' come to mind. It is often accompanied by a *thudding heartbeat and sometimes a hot flush*. It normally stops when I get up. However, it then produces another set of symptoms which often persist throughout the day and last over several days.

Again I struggle for words, but it is as if there is a continuous upward pressure from my diaphragm, under my ribcage – 'uptight' springs to mind. I have the feeling one gets from holding one's breath, though I appear to be breathing normally. The best relief, albeit very shortlived, comes from a deep breath, or particularly from a yawn. In these conditions I yawn prodigiously which can be embarrassing in company! It is not a pain, though is often a persistent ache in the diaphragm which sometimes spreads through to my back and shoulders. It lasts for days or even weeks and makes me feel very tired, irritable and depressed.

Comment There is, not surprisingly, no clear explanation for these 'horrible' sensations – though the pounding heart in the second of these descriptions from Mrs M.J. is suggestive of some generalized arousal of the autonomic nervous system as described by another reader, Mrs P.E. from Croydon, in the section on chest pain. This description also has some features in common with one of the Kundalini experiences in the immediately preceding section, where a 'hot explosion sends painful tingles through the chest, abdomen and down both arms'.

The most thorough investigations failed to produce a positive diagnosis, but the following possibilities have been suggested.

Sleep Apnoea

This curious condition, where heavy snorers intermittently stop breathing (apnoea) throughout the night leading to the accumulation of carbon dioxide in the blood, has been implicated. 'I am almost sure these symptoms are caused by breath-holding which happens when I have been very worried or having a nightmare. I have done this occasionally and woken in an awful panic with a feeling of distress – breathing deeply of course puts it right.'

Panic Attacks

Panic attacks associated with unpleasant dreams may also be an answer: 'I started to have panic attacks and feelings of pressure in my chest when I started the menopause. They would usually be preceded by a very unpleasant anxiety dream.'

Beta blockers

'I too had some sort of panic sensation and rapid heartbeat on waking in the night when, before being fully conscious, I had a sensation of *swelling of "bubbles" in the bloodstream*. Eventually my doctor prescribed the beta blocker half-inderal LA.

I only need to take six and the whole problem disappears. I still occasionally have to take perhaps one a week just to clear up any slight jitteriness or nervousness – but they work very well and I recommend them.'

Morbid Thoughts

It is interesting to note how morbid thoughts seem to occur most frequently in the early morning after waking and these may give rise to this type of physical symptoms. These morbid thoughts can be controlled, as Mr H.R. from France writes:

For many years I was assailed, mostly on first awakening, with what I could describe as a melancholy which moved round easily into a wretched state of depression. It would slowly lift as the day progressed and I would wonder why this happened. About a year ago I realized how readily I was content to give my full attention to any idea that came to me and when – as often it was – on the dark side I would feed it to the point when thoughts such as 'What am I doing in this life?' would have full reign. Black stuff indeed. The recognition in understanding what I was doing in creating this mind set was truly a turning point. I did an about-turn and switched off the negative thoughts. From that time I have had total freedom from this demon.

PAINFUL NOCTURNAL ERECTIONS

Query 66-year-old Mr J.R. of Cambridgeshire writes:

For the last 15 years I have woken twice in the night at exactly 3.40 a.m. and 6.00 a.m. with an erection, violent gurgling stomach and churning testicles. On rising for breakfast I start to feel dreadful and with a sense of foreboding. This is no normal early morning erection and has continued in varying intensity for 13 years. I have been unable to find any relief from this involuntary condition, or anyone with similar symptoms.

Comment This syndrome of sleep-related painful erections has been investigated by Dr B.J. Matthews of London's Atkinson Morley Hospital, who describes a further case in a 63-year-old man.

This gentleman was referred to our laboratory with a 20-year history of repeated wakenings at night by painful erections. These were different in quality compared with his normal erections, being very rigid and associated with a feeling of pressure in his perineum. Most nights he wakened with them on at least four occasions, went to the toilet to pass water, lost the erection and returned to sleep. He was increasingly dissatisfied with his sleep and was tense and irritable during the day. Often he noted he had been dreaming when he wakened. He experienced normal erections at other times, which caused him no discomfort and his sexual relationship was fairly satisfactory.

The symptoms began a few years before his marriage at the age of 43, initially very irregularly. Gradually they worsened, but urological surgeons found no explanation after intensive investigations. Mild symptoms of anxiety and depression led to a referral for a psychiatric assessment, but neither the treatment with anti-depressants nor psychotherapy were of any benefit.

We initiated treatment with 10mg of Propranolol at night which intially completely abolished his symptoms. His sexual function remained normal and although erections occurred at night they lost their painful quality. However, after three months the symptoms gradually returned. With an increase in dosage his similar but faster habituation recurred. At present his symptoms are still uncontrolled.

NODDING OFF – THE OPERA SYNDROME

Query Mr J.D. from London writes:

Two friends of mine, both male and in their mid-30s, have experienced the same problem. *When they go with me and other friends to the opera or theatre they find they tend to become drowsy and fall asleep about 15 minutes after the performance starts*. When they wake up (or more frequently are nudged awake) the problem seems to go away – although I have to say it does need continuous nudging and kicking to do so. Both are quite lively before the performance and after the nap can keep going until the early hours of the morning. I wonder if it has anything to do with the effect on the eyes of the auditorium lights going down because the same thing does not happen in a concert hall whose lights are not usually reduced as much as at the theatre or opera.

Comment There were two suggestions as to how to overcome this unfortunate habit, made the more irritating by the cost of a night out at the opera.

(i) *Afternoon nap*: 'As soon as I enter the theatre or opera house and the lights dim I am away – into deep sleep. It is maddening to be "out for the count" within five minutes. I too am lively before curtain up and keep going after. My own diagnosis is that this occurs because of the strong similarity between going to bed – into a snug environment, lights out (or dimmed) and the excitements of the day catch up and put you into sleep. The only preventative measure to take is an afternoon nap – in bed, in a darkened room.'

(ii) *Deep yawn*: 'My suggestion to overcome this problem is to take three slow deep breaths and keep repeating until the sleep dissolves.'

There are several further sleep-related mystery syndromes which do not really fit into any of the categories mentioned above.

ELECTRIC SHOCKS TO LEGS

Query Mrs P.J. from Kent writes:

About two hours after falling asleep I wake – usually after a mildly disturbing dream – to *an awful sensation in my legs. It can best be described as an electric shock. I feel every nerve is standing on edge.* The only relief is to rub downwards. It sometimes makes me cry and as all fears seem to be magnified in the small hours, I can't help wondering about 'spontaneous combustion'. My doctor does not seem to take it seriously. Her attitude could be summed up as 'amused incredulity' – but I assure you I do not find it funny.

TIGHT HEAD AND NAUSEA

Query Mrs S.M. from Sutton Coldfield writes:

I am getting desperate as I can't get any refreshing sleep. I get plenty of sleep in quantity but not quality. *I wake up several times after a vivid dream with a tight head and nausea and weakness in my limbs.* This happens throughout the night until eventually I wake up in the morning exhausted and have a terrible day – not being able to do much or communicate with anyone, go to bed and it all starts all over again.

DRY MOUTH

Query Mr C.J. from Lancashire writes:

Initially it began with *dryness in the mouth during the night, causing me to wake several times and drink water.* In 18 months it has been preceded by *intense dreaming.* If I do not rise early, say around 5.00 a.m., the head pains and backache occur. Sleep seems to be the trigger of my symptoms as they do not occur in the daytime unless I nap in the afternoon.

POUNDING HEAD AND PROFUSE SWEATING

Query Mr W.J. from Kent writes:

For the past ten years I have had a particular health problem whose symptoms have not changed. I go to bed at night feeling upbeat. I go to sleep immediately. After about four hours I wake with some slight reflux. I have a distinct pounding in my head and a strong (but not racing) pulse. I have been sweating profusely and my hair around the nape of my neck is wet. I need to change my pyjama jacket. Next day I have a headache and distinct lethargy. I have had massive doses of the acid-suppressant drug Losec, but still I get the symptoms.

18
A Clutch of Curiosities

This concluding section features a clutch of curiosities, ranging from tweaky bum to flat beer syndrome that do not readily fit into any of the categories already considered.

'TWEAKY BUM'

Query 64-year-old Mr P.D. from Worthing writes: '*Whenever I witness a painful incident or even just hear somebody describing a major operation or a slight accident – I sustain a quite severe pain in my rectum.* I have never thought of myself as being squeamish and I am mystified by this reaction to events.'

Comment It is possible that this pain is similar to that of proctalgia fugax (see Chapter 9, Rectal Pain) brought on by spasm of the anal muscle in response to sudden tension. A 56-year-old male reader from Yorkshire observes: 'It is most notable when watching television – whenever I see someone fall in such a way as to cause considerable pain, I feel a tightening and pain in my rectum which coincides with the event – such that it is as if I am experiencing the same fall.'

There also seems to be a genetic element, as it runs in families.

♦ 'All our family are familiar with this response, although the pain is not exactly severe. We joked about it when the children were young and were all aware of it when looking over a precipice such as a high wall or from cliffs overlooking the sea. We call it "tweaky bum", which is hardly elegant – but describes the feeling well.'

The sensation, however, is not necessarily confined to the rectum, as the following two comments make clear:

♦ 'All my life I have experienced painful experiences in both my legs whenever I witness or hear of an accident or major operation, or similar traumatic happening. I have never met anyone with the same sensation.'

♦ 'I had an above-the-knee amputation 52 years ago, and ever since I have suffered periods of intense nerve pains in the missing leg, not unlike electric shock. During the time when I am not experiencing this pain, I only have to think of some trauma – such as seeing my wife using a sharp knife, carving dangerously, or observing a near accident when out walking, to have one of these "shocks" which are so severe I have difficulty in not calling out.

Treatment The only suggested 'cure' for tweaky bum turned out to be quite drastic:

(i) 'I do suffer pain in the rectum when hearing or reading about blood curdling or traumatic events. The cure came unexpectedly when I had a colonic resection of a cancer some years later. My body has settled down nicely with its rerouted exit system and I do not have the slightest twinge when hearing or reading about even the most spine-chilling disasters.

DISTANT PAIN (OR ITCH)

Query Mr J.M. from Stockport writes: 'I have been experiencing *severe shooting pains down my left leg*, without warning, that stop me completely. The pain disappears as quickly as it came. One day I noticed that it sometimes started as I put my hat on which was rather surprising until I realized that touching the top of my left ear precipitated the spasm.'

Comment A similar phenomenon has been reported in the *New Scientist*:

> Recently I had an itch on my right forearm. I scratched it hard with a sharp left fingernail. In experiencing the usual momentary ecstasty of an itch well scratched, I concurrently felt the *stabbing pain just above the waistline at the left side of my back*. The more vigorously I scratched my arm, the more intensely I felt the sympathetic stabbing in my back. Several days later I found the scab I had created on my arm and attacked it again – and found that the exact same point on my lower left back was being stabbed once more. Why?'

Professor P.K. Thomas, formerly of the Institute of Neurology in London, observes:

> This is a not uncommon phenomenon, known as referred itch (or pain), or *Mitempfindungen* (from the German *mitempfinden*, which means 'to sympathize with'). It was first described by the Reverend Steven Hales, an English cleric and experimental physiologist, back in 1773. The mechanism is not established, but the sensation is probably transmitted by fibre tracks within the spinal cord and is dependent upon temporary changes in nerve cell excitability.

It is possible that the pins and needles experienced in the hands on urination described in Chapter 11 may be a manifestation of this phenomenon.

MUSIC-INDUCED TICKLE

Query Mrs C.P. from Derby writes: '*There are certain pieces of piano music which, if I play, produce a sneezy tickle on the bridge of my nose!* Even if I don't play this particular piece for a year, whenever I put the music in front of me and begin to play, the sneezy tickle comes and perseveres until the end. The little piece of music is Grieg's "Springtanz Opus 17".'

Comment There are three explanations for this bizarre phenomenon.

Allergy

It is possible that a chemical substance emanating from the printed copy of the music may be responsible. One way of testing this would be to play this piece of music wearing a gas mask which, as one reader observed, is not as absurd as it might seem. During the war, numerous keyboard addicts would confidently reach for their gas masks before practising passages *fortissimo*, which through concentration and sheer volume of sound, might render the siren sounds unheard – leaving them susceptible to gas and its dire consequences.

Musical Vibration

The nose distinguishes smell based on the specific vibration of the substance with which it comes into contact. If, for example, a substance vibrated at 3.5K per second, the specific response would be recorded by the brain. Even if one reproduces this vibration without the substance, one still smelt it. Could it be that certain vibrations from Grieg's 'Springtanz Opus 17' vibrate in a similar way to a substance which might cause a sneeze sensation?

Epilepsy

It is possible that this sneezy tickle is a benign variety of epilepsy – a well-recognized phenomenon in which specific notes can trigger an electrical discharge within the brain. This usually causes an 'absence' or fit, but can produce virtually any neurological symptoms, giddiness, pins and needles and perhaps even a sneezing tickle.

MIGRATING SKIN SENSITIVITY

Mrs D.E. from North London writes:

It all started with flu-like symptoms and tiredness, which then progressed to sensitivity of the skin (with itching and pain) on different parts of the body – thighs, armpits, back of upper arms, shoulders, midriff, just below the rib cage. *The sensitivity remained in one area for a few weeks before moving on to another area.* The sensitivity is to *light touch only.* Heavy pressure has no effect, in fact gives relief. Light brushing of clothes against the sensitive *areas* when moving about is worse. This in turn sets off shivery feelings, flu like symptoms and feelings of fatigue, especially in the evening. The only recourse is to go to bed.

Comment This syndrome remains unexplained, though the shifting site of the sensitive skin is similar to the condition known as Wartenberg's neuritis. This is brought on by stretching of the sensory nerves under the skin, resulting in pain and numbness, as another reader describes:

There is no warning, as a gentle stretch can bring on a feeling of of the tearing of the peripheral nerves under the skin as if being flayed or burned. The pain is acute momentarily – but once it has taken place, the pain dies away, only to return each time the same stretch is repeated. It gradually lessens over time and can take anything from six months to a year to heal. Meanwhile there is a central area of numbness from which the soreness radiates. When one area eventually returns to normal another area takes over. Pressing the area has no effect, but gentle stretching can be excruciating.

Dr W.B. Mathews of Oxford's Radcliffe Infirmary describes the case of a 62-year-old male doctor, who had experienced these symptoms for 30 years:

It was originally limited to the index finger of both hands. At first the sequence of pain on stretching leading to numbness continued unchanged – but after repeated episodes slight alterations of perception persisted in that area for many months. Around the age of 55, the skin on the lower limbs began to be affected, at one time producing symmetrical patches of numbness between the patella and the head of the fibula. Kneeling while gardening was the usual cause of the stretch and again sensory change, amounting to no more than slight sensitivity to touch, became persistent.

REPETITIVE TUNE SYNDROME

Mrs G.L. from Surrey writes: 'I suffer from what in modern parlance would be called repetitive tune syndrome. *A song or piece of music comes into my mind and repeats itself through-out the day however much one tries to dismiss it.* Several people I know experience this and although it is not an ailment it is highly irritating.'

Comment Many readers described a similar experience:

- ◆ 'A tune is constantly going on in my head and is particu-larly obtrusive when reading. Sometimes it goes on when I am actually listening to other music; the result can be very discordant.'
- ◆ 'It is not just isolated tunes but whole passages of sym-phonies that enter my brain out of the blue and repeat themselves endlessly. They may be compositions I have heard weeks or even months previously. I hear them completely intact – each instrument playing its part and in perfect pitch.'

Treatment The solution would seem to be to replace the intru-sive melody deliberately with another.

(i) 'My father used to sing "Onward Christian Soldiers" at the top of his splendid voice to dislodge a tune in the brain. It expressed sentiments he believed in wholeheartedly.'
(ii) 'The "Sky Boat Song" will eradicate an irritating tune. Then itself fades away.'

TRAVEL PHOBIA

Mr R.W. from Bristol writes:

> I am 69 and for the past ten years *have become increasingly reluctant to take holidays or indeed to stay away at all.* I have noticed similar behaviour in a number of men in my age group – men who when younger grabbed every chance they could to travel. I myself in my 20s gave up a job I loved to go and work in a construction camp on Vancouver Island for a year. It is throwing rather a strain on my marriage.

Comment There are several observations, of varying degrees of sympathy, on this gentleman's plight.

♦ 'My husband spent his working life travelling all over the world and he enjoyed foreign holidays very much. He was 57 when he quite suddenly refused to travel abroad. Now at 66 he is reluctant to leave the village for a night away yet alone a weekend. He is perfectly happy and enjoys a good social life. I found it difficult at first but have come to terms with holidays alone and our family always visit us. On reflection his father was almost exactly the same – maybe it is inherited.'

♦ 'Your correspondent has clearly acquired the wisdom to appreciate that the inconvenience and expense of moving his body from place A to place B to no good or profitable purpose is an exercise in sheer futility. No blame can be attached to his wife for her failure to share this pragmatism, but the issue arises simply as a result of the genetic difference between the sexes. The answer is to allow one's wife a degree of independence. Mine for instance took a holiday in Australia by herself last year.'

♦ 'This is male egotistical ego syndrome. The answer is simple – go on holidays with girlfriends and relations or alone. Do exactly what you want to for a fortnight. Come back and your husband is really pleased to see you.'

SUMMER BLUES

Query Mr G.H. from Bristol writes:

I feel at my best in the winter months. *I feel 'under the weather' from some time in the summer until early October. During my 'bad' months I feel my energy draining after walking about a mile.* I feel so weak I have to rest. In these months I feel low and often depressed. Everything is too much bother to do. In October I revert to normal and once again feel fit and well.

Comment This is known as reverse Seasonal Affective Disorder, or reverse SAD being the precise opposite of the usual presentation of SAD, when depression lasts throughout the winter months only to disappear at the advent of summer. Another reader comments:

> I too suffer from reverse SAD and would like to be able to hibernate throughout July and August and wake up when cooler temperatures return. I am not saying I 'like' the extra hours of darkness in the winter but it is a small price to pay in return for cooler temperatures. In spring, autumn and winter I am a busy and happy 57-year-old, but as soon as the temperature approaches 70°F I am a worn-out old crock.

Dr Thomas Wehr of the National Institute of Mental Health in America describes a further case:

> Mr B., a 45-year-old married professor, was energetic, ambitious and enthusiastic – but had marked difficulty in functioning because of depression in the summer months in southern climates. These summer depressions had begun in childhood when he had lived near the Mediterranean. In Northern Europe and New England he had little difficulty in summer. When he was in his mid-30s, he moved to Washington DC and again had severe depressions in the summer. For the next eight years he was treated every summer with antidepressants, which were beneficial.

There was also a suggestion that it might be due to sleep deprivation: 'In winter the sufferer probably gets a full night's sleep and therefore has plenty of daytime energy. However, as the nights shorten, the sleeping hours tend to lessen and the rejuvenation that sleep brings becomes less. This is nature's way – the old saying, up with the lark.'

The obvious remedy here is to fit blackout linings to bedroom curtains and have a short nap after lunch!

Treatment Several readers recommend the antidepressant natural remedy St John's wort as helpful, and another observed, 'I found that taking coenzyme QT 20mg a day was helpful – but I should love to find a way of coping with the feeling of heaviness in my limbs and the mental inertia which accompanies it, particularly as I like to take part in various summer activities with my two small grandsons.'

NECK SPASM AND DRAMATIC CHANGE IN MOOD

Query Mr B.S. from Surrey writes:

My mood can change dramatically within seconds and is all linked to what feels like a muscle spasm at the point where the spine 'meets' the head. If the point of pressure moves by a very small distance I feel released and can lead a normal life and feel fine! If it doesn't move I can spend a day feeling totally miserable and having no interest in anything and feeling very detached and foggy. It is worse when lying down or when I place my head on a pillow so sleep is impaired, but it improves rapidly within the first 30 minutes of being awake.

Comment There are two other very similar descriptions of the same phenomenon:

♦ 'I have a very similar condition. Either my neck is as it should be and I am happy, or it is "out" and I am utterly miseable. It has been "out" now for three months and six trips to an osteopath have not helped.'

♦ 'My neck and head seem to be permanently "touchy", starting from the top of my neck with various aches, pressure tightness and prickly feelings over the head, face and neck. Some days my moods are on a short fuse and seem to be connected to muscle spasm sensations or sharp pains in the back of the head. I have had physiotherapy, acupuncture, cortisone injections, MRI scans and tried the usual things, special-shaped pillows, aromatherapy oils etc.'

This syndrome is very perplexing, but the following comments are of interest:

Every chiropractor I have talked to on the subject knows that a 'subluxation' (slightly out of position) of the joint at the top of the neck is linked to psychological states of mind. My advice is to stop doing any exercises his osteopath might have given him and let his spine settle down and stiffen up. In time he should consult a chiropracter who will position the joint correctly without overmobilizing it. This should alleviate the spasms.

FLAT BEER SYNDROME

Query Mr G.T. from Oxford writes:

When I drink a pint of beer it goes flat in the glass immediately. When the glass is refilled the beer immediately loses its head – even before I have touched it. It seems I must have left some chemical in the glass which has this effect. I would not be over concerned, but I have also been feeling very tired and suffering from dizzy spells, chest pains and muscle spasms. My urine is frequently oily. It has been tested and nothing has been found. I also note that if I drink red wine an oily film forms on the top.

Comment Several readers comment on a similar experience.

♦ 'We like a bit of froth on our beer in these northern parts. Many years ago I knew a pub landlady who could tell when a drinker had had a fatty meal like a pork chop or anything fried. How? When he took the first sip of the pint of beer she had just pulled, the froth disappeared.'

♦ 'I usually have a glass of lager during the evening but as I don't like cold drinks I don't chill the can, resulting in a large head. Purely by chance I found that dipping a greasy knife blade into the froth caused it to condense into large bubbles and disappear, leaving no head.'

♦ 'I noticed at school that if you took a sip of soup that was too hot and rejected it into the bowl – the soup shortly became more runny. My assumption was that something in the saliva had interacted with the soup.'

♦ 'Several years ago some friends and I in the local pub on Sunday lunchtime noticed the odd person's beer would go flat for no apparent reason and if the glass was refilled it would go flat. Over a period of time we worked out and then proved that if we had fried food for breakfast or within a few hours, the beer would go flat.'

♦ 'A layer of grease acts as an "anti-foaming agent" so residual grease in the glass or residues of washing up liquid also destroy the foam.'

So it would appear that Mr G.T.'s saliva has a high concentration of some enzyme in it, probably amylase, which is responsible for this effect.

Some 30 years ago I had a friend with the same problem – the moment his lips touched the glass any head on his pint of real ale disappeared. Further, as he worked his way down the glass there was never a tidemark of froth left after each draught.

He happened to mention this to his dentist on one of his rare visits and was told this was caused by a very high concentration of an enzyme in his saliva, which also had the sublime advantage of killing almost all decay-causing substances. As my friend was rising 40 and didn't have a filling in his head, this struck me as entirely plausible.

References

2: THE SENSE ORGANS: EYES, EARS, NOSE AND MOUTH

The Eyes

F. Quaranta Leoni, 'Strategies for managing watering eyes', *The Practitioner* 1997: 241; 182–4

Mark Wright, 'Diagnosis and treatment of dry eye', *The Practitioner* 1997: 241; 210–14

J. Pearce, 'What's in a name: The needle in the eye syndrome', *World Medicine* 1979: Jan 13; 77–9

Brian Ellis, 'Referred ocular pain relieved by suboccipital injection', *Headache* 1995: 35; 101–3

David Coulter, 'Eye pain with nifedipine', *British Medical Journal* 1988: 246; 1086–8

V.M. Reading, 'Eye strain and visual display units', *The Lancet* 1986: 1; 905

M.A. Rosenblat, 'Ocular and periocular pain', *Otolaryngologic Clinics of North America* 1989: 22; 1173–203

The Ears

T. Lamer, 'Ear pain due to cervical spine arthritis', *Headache* 1991: 11;155–7

J. Costen, 'A syndrome of ear and sinus symptoms dependent upon disturbed function of the temporomandibular joint', *Ann Otol Rhinol Laryngol* 1997: 106; 805–19

J.N. Blau, 'Ear pain referred by the vagus', *British Medical Journal* 1999: 299; 1569–70

S. Metzger, 'Chondrodermatitis helicis chronica: A clinical re-evaluation and pathological review', *The Laryngoscope* 1975: 1402–11.

The Nose

J.W. Georgitis, 'Ipatropium bromide nasal spray in non-allergic rhinitis', *Clinical and Experimenal Allergy* 1994: 24; 1049–55

M.J. Brockbank, 'Cerebro spinal fluid in the rhinitis clinic', *The Journal of Laryngology and Otology* 1989: 103; 281–3

J. Nuutinen, 'Balanced physiological saline in the treatment of chronic rhinitis', *Rhinology* 1986: 24; 265–9

The Mouth

P.J. Lamey, 'Burning mouth syndrome', *Dental Update* September 1998: 298–300

U.F. Hulstein, 'Burning mouth syndrome due to nicotinic acid, esters and sorbic acid', *Contact Dermatitis* 1988: 19; 225–6

M. Garcis-Bravatti, 'Burning mouth syndrome', *American Journal of Gastroenterology* 1996: 91; 1281

W. Huang, 'The burning mouth syndrome', *Journal of the American Academy of Dermatology* 1996: 34; 92–6

G. Humphris, 'Cognitive therapy for burning mouth syndrome', *British Dental Journal* 1996: 181; 204–8

Frank Powell, 'Glossodynia and other disorders of the tongue', *Dermatologic Clinics* 1987: 5; 687–90

D.A. Dresner, 'Geographic tongue', *Otolaryngology – Head and Neck Surgery* 1997: 117; 291

J.A. Langtry, 'Topical tretinoin: a new treatment for black hairy tongue', *Clinical and Experimental Dermatology* 1992: 17; 163–4

R.A. Thompson, 'Response of "idiopathic" recurrent angioneurotic oedema to tranexamic acid', *British Medical Journal* 1978 26 August, p. 608

Brian Johnston, 'Swallowing and oesophageal function in Parkinson's Disease', *American Journal of Gastroenterology* 1995: 90; 1741–6

Martin Burton, 'The surgical management of drooling', *Developmental Medicine and Child Neurology* 1991: 33; 1110–16

D. Readihough, 'Use of benzhexol hydrochloride to control drooling of children with cerebral palsy', *Developmental Medicine and Child Neurology* 1990: 32; 985–9

B.K. Young, 'Surgical management of drooling', *Australian Dental Journal* 1992: 37; 115

I. Watanabe, 'Oral dyskinesia of the aged', *Gerodontics* 1985: 1; 39–43. *Gerodontics* 1988: 4; 310–4

E. Vager, 'Prevalence of spontaneous oral dyskinesia in the elderly', *American Journal of Psychiatry* 1982: 139; 1329–31

Howard Suture, 'Oro-facial dyskinesia: A dental dimension', *JAMA* 1971: 216; 1459–62

G. Sedman, 'Clonazepam in treatment of oral dyskinesia', *British Medical Journal* 1976, 4 September; 58

L. Reik, 'Atypical odontalgia', *Headache* 1984: 5; 222–6

Rollin Gallagher, 'Chronic pain', *The Medical Clinics of North America* 1999: 83; 700–5

R. Czerninsky, 'Odontalgia in vascular oro-facial pain', *Journal of Oro-facial Pain* 1999: 13; 196–200

3: THE SENSES: VISION, HEARING, TASTE AND SMELL

Vision

G.P.S. Barodawla, 'Visual hallucinations', *Journal of the Royal College of Physicians of London* 1997: 31; 42–7

N.J. White, 'Complex visual hallucinations in partial blindness due to eye disease', *British Journal of Psychiatry* 1980: 136; 284–6

George W. Paulson, 'Visual hallucinations in the elderly', *Gerontology* 1997: 43; 255–60

W. Dewi Rees, 'The hallucinations of widowhood', *British Medical Journal* 1971 2 October, 33–41

Kenneth Gold, 'Isolated visual hallucinations and the Charles Bonnet syndrome', *Comprehensive Psychiatry* 1989: 30; 92–7

David Smith, 'Micropsia', *Clinical Paediatrics* 1980: 19; 297–9

Stuart Copperman, 'Alice in Wonderland Syndrome as a presenting symptom of infectious mononucleosis in children', *Clinical Paediatrics* 1977: 16; 143–150

Gerald Golden, 'The Alice in Wonderland Syndrome in juvenile migraine', *Clinical Paediatrics* 1979: 63; 517–19

Hearing

Gunther Deutschel, 'Ear click in palatal tremor', *Neurology* 1991: 41: 1677–9

P. Vieregge, 'The diagnosis of "essential palatal tremor" ', *Neurology* 1997: 49; 248–9

Taste and Smell

Allan Knight, 'Anosmia', *The Lancet* 1988: ii; 512

R.I. Henkin, 'Disordered smell', *The Lancet* 1988: ii; 902

R.I. Henkin, 'Salty and bitter taste', *JAMA* 1991: 265; 225

R.I. Henkin, 'Idiopathic hypogeusia', *JAMA* 1971: 217; 434–40

Daniel Deames, 'Spontaneous resolution of dysgeusia', *Arch Otolaryngol Head Neck Surgery* 1996: 122; 961–3

Christine Lawrence, 'Dysgeusia', *The Lancet* 1996: 348; 1102

Albert Freedman, 'Taste for zinc', *The Lancet* 1996: 348; 1592

B.H. Ackerman, 'Disturbances of taste and smell induced by drugs', *Pharmacotherapy* 1997: 17; 482–96

4: HEADACHE

N. Fox, 'A communication headache', *British Medical Journal* 1999: 318; 802

L. Newman, 'Hemicrania continua', *Neurology* 1994: 44; 211–15

L. Newman, 'Hypnic head syndrome: A benign headache disorder of the elderly', *Neurology* 1990: 40; 1904

E. Martin, 'Cephalgia fugax: A momentary headache', *British Medical Journal* 1986: 292; 663–4

N. Raskin, 'Icepick-like pain', *Neurology* 1980: 30; 203–5

M. Porter, 'Benign coital cephalgia', *Arch Neurology* 1981: 38; 710–11

B. Williams, 'Cough headache due to craniospinal pressure dissociation, 1980: 37; 226–9

G. Gilbert, 'Hypoxia and bedcovers', *JAMA* 1972: 221; 1165–6

J. Pearce, 'Exploding head syndrome', *The Lancet* 1988: 2; 68

5: FACIAL PAIN

Charlotte Feinmann, *The Mouth, the Face and the Mind* OUP 1999

S.B. Graff-Radford, 'Facial pain', *Current Opinion in Neurology* 2000: 13; 291–6

S.C. Pannullo, 'Trigeminal neuralgia – neurosurgical management options', *Journal of the American Dental Association* 1996: 127; 1635–9

J.K. Campbell, 'Facial pain due to migraine and cluster headaches', *Seminars in Neurology* 1988: 8; 324–31

C. Hansen, 'Treatment of chronic pain with anti-epileptic drugs: a new era', *Southern Medical Journal* 1999: 92; 642–8

6: VERTIGO AND COLLAPSE

K. Kroenke, 'How common are various causes of dizziness?' *Southern Medical Journal* 2000: 93; 160–7

J.E. Isaacson, 'Otolaryngologic management of dizziness in the older patient', *Clinics in Geriatric Medicine* 1999: 15; 179–91

R.W. Baloh, 'Vertigo', *The Lancet* 1998: 352; 1841–6

G.D. Johnson, 'Medical Management of Migraine related dizziness in vertigo', *Laryngoscope* 1998: 108; 1–18

Michael Cutrer, 'Migraine-associated dizziness', *Headache* 1992: 32; 300–4

D. Bradley Welling, 'Particle repositioning manoeuvre for benign paroxysmal positional vertigo', *Laryngoscope* 1994: 104; 946–8

T. Lempert, 'Benign positional vertigo', *British Medical Journal* 1995: 311; 489–91

G.M.S. Ryan, 'Cervical vertigo', *The Lancet* 1955: 2; 1355–7

A.B. Dey, 'Drop attacks in the elderly revisited', *Quarterly Journal of Medicine* 1997: 90; 1–3

Myung Sic L. Lee, 'Drop attacks' *Advances in Neurology* 1995: 67; 41–53

D.L. Stevens, 'Cryptogenic drop attacks: An affliction of women?' *British Medical Journal* 1973: 24 February; 439–43

Irene Meissner, 'The natural history of drop attacks', *Neurology* 1986: 36; 1029–34

A.B. Dey, 'Cardiovascular syncopy is the most common cause of drop attacks in the elderly', *Pace* 1997: 20; 818–19

B. Olshansky, 'A Pepsi Challenge', *NEJM* 1999: 340; 2006

G.J. Norel, 'Drop attacks and instability of the cervical spine', *Journal of Bone and Joint Surgery* 1996: 78; 465–6

7: THROAT AND VOICE

Nathan Pearlman, 'Primary upper aerodigestive tract manifestations of gastro-oesophageal reflux', *American Journal of Gastroenterology* 1988: 83; 22–4

Stephen Schaefer, 'Spasmodic dysphonia', *Otolaryngologic Clinics of North America* 1987: 20; 161–75

Adrian Williams, 'Consensus statement for the management of focal dystonias', *British Journal of Hospital Medicine* 1993: 50; 655–8

R.H. Miller, 'Treatment options in spasmodic dysphonia', *Otolaryngologic Clinics of North America* 1991: 24; 1227–37

J.K. Casper, 'Voice therapy methods in dysphonia', *Otolaryngologic Clinics of North America* 2000: 33; 983–1002

S.R. Gibbs, 'Botulinum toxin for the treatment of spasmodic dysphonia', *Otolaryngologic Clinics of North America* 2000: 33; 879–94

David Krohn, 'A study of the effectiveness of a specific treatment for elective mutism,' *Journal of the American Academy of Child Adolescent Psychiatry* 1992: 31; 711–17

Bruce Black, 'Treatment of elective mutism with fluoxetine', *Journal of the American Academy of Child Adolescent Psychiatry* 1994: 33

8: THE CHEST

G. Lanza, 'Angina pectoris and headache', *The Lancet* 2000: 356; 998

M. Moren Bryhn, 'Ear pain due to myocardial ischaemia', *American Heart Journal* 107; 1

Gerald Levey, 'Tietze's Syndrome', *Arthritis and Rheumatism* 1962: 5; 261–7

Adele Fam, 'Musculo-skeletal chest wall pain', *Cambridge Medical Association Journal* 1985: 133; 379–380

Eliot Semble, 'Chest pain: A Rheumatologist's Perspective', *Southern Medical Journal* 1988: 81

Robert Reichstein, 'Nasal pruritus as atypical angina', *New England Journal of Medicine* 309; 667

K.F. Chung, 'Diagnosis and management of chronic persistent dry cough', *Postgraduate Medical Journal* 1996: 72; 595–8

Paul Glasziou, 'Twenty-year cough in a non-smoker', *British Medical Journal* 1998: vol. 316; 1660–1

John Vane, 'Trumping the ace', *The Lancet* 1995: vol. 346; 916

K.O. Paulose, 'Otogenic reflex cough: Implanted hair in the bony external auditory canal', *Arch Otolaryngol Head and Neck Surgery* 1988: vol. 114; 1234

Majed Odeh, 'A man who coughed for 15 years before a doctor took his pulse', *The Lancet* 1996: vol. 348; 378

Jonathan Abrams, 'Nocturnal palpitations', *JAMA* 1987: 257; 1961

B. Hill Britton, 'Pulsatile tinnitus not nocturnal palpitations', *JAMA* 1987: 258; 779

M. Leonhardt, 'Pathological yawning associated with periodic leg movements in sleep: cured by Levodopa', *Journal of Neurology* 1999: 2; 621–2

B. Van Sweden, 'Excessive yawning', *Acta Neurologica Belgica* 1994: 150–1; 494

H. Wimalaratna, 'Is yawning a brain stem phenomenon?', *The Lancet* 1988: 1; 300

9: THE GUT

Editorial, 'Management of diffuse oesophageal spasm', *The Lancet* 1987: I; 80

Salah Nasrallah, 'Nifedipine in the treatment of diffuse oesophageal spasm', *The Lancet* 1982: II; 1284

James Helm, 'Salivary responses to oesophageal acid in normal subjects and patients with reflux', *Gastroenterology* 1987: 93; 1393–7

J.P. Drenth, 'Efficacy of diltiazem in the treatment of diffuse oesophageal spasm', *Alimentary Pharmacology and Therapeutics* 1990: 4; 411–6

N.J. Talley, 'Functional gastroduodenal disorders', *Gut* 1999: 45(SII); 37–42

H. Mertz, 'Symptoms and visceral perception in severe functional and organic dyspepsia', *Gut* 1998: 42; 814–22

Fernando Cervero, 'Visceral hyperalgesia revisited', *The Lancet* 2000: 356; 1127–8

P.G. Farup, 'Ranitidine effectively relieves symptoms in a subset of patients with functional dyspepsia', *Scandinavian Journal of Gastroenterology* 1997: 32; 755–9

H.J. Son, 'Hypersensitivity to acid in ulcer-like functional dyspepsia', *Korean Journal of Internal Medicine* 1997: 12; 188–92

Dr A.T.R. Axon, 'Abdominal migraine – does it exist?', *Journal of Clinical Gastroenterology* 1991: 13; 615–6

J.N. Blau, 'Is abdominal pain a feature of adult migraine?' *Headache* 1995: 35; 207–9

J.A. Moran, 'Adult abdominal migraine and sumatriptan', *Irish Medical Journal* 1998: 91; 215–6

Dr D.E. Long, 'Abdominal migraine: cause of abdominal pain in adults', *Journal of Gastroenterology and Hepatology* 1992: 7; 210–13

David Symon, 'Double blind placebo controlled trial of Pizotifen in the treatment of abdominal migraine', *Archives of Diseases of Childhood* 1995: 72; 48–50

D. Bentley, 'Abdominal migraine and food sensitivity in children', *Clinical Allergy* 1984: 14; 499–500

W. Grant Thompson, 'Proctalgia fugax', *Journal of the Royal College of Physicians* 1980: 14; 247–8

'Anal neuralgia', *The Lancet* 1931: 2; 877

J.E. Wright, 'Inhaled salbutamol for proctalgia fugax', *The Lancet* 1985: 1; 659–60

Richard Duggan, 'Familial rectal pain', *The Lancet* 1972: 1; 854

Romaine Schubert, 'Familial Rectal Pain', *The Annals of Neurology* 1992: 32; 824–6

John Bascom, 'Pudendal canal syndrome and proctalgia fugax', *Dis Col Rectum* March 1998; 406

Neil Hagen, 'Sharp shooting neuropathic pain in the rectum or genitals: pudendal neuralgia', *Journal of Pain and Symptom Management* 1993: 7; 496–500

Linda Frazier, 'Coccydynia: a tale of woe', *North Carolina Medical Journal* 1985: 46; 209–12

Christopher Wray, 'Coccydynia', *Journal of Bone and Joint Surgery* 1991: 73; 335–8

Stuart Grant, 'Levator Syndrome', *Dis Col Rectum* 1975: 18; 161–3

10: SMELLS

R. Ayesh, 'Body malodour syndromes', *The Lancet* 1995: 345; 1308

Michelle Smith, 'The use of smell in differential diagnosis', *The Lancet* 1982: 2; 1452

Thomas Cone, 'Diagnosis and treatment: some diseases, syndromes and conditions associated with an unusual odour', *Paediatrics* 1968: 41; 993–5

Irvine Golding, 'An unusual case of bromidrosis', *Paediatrics* 1965: 36; 791–2

Peter Molberg, 'Body odour from topical benzoyl peroxide', *New England Journal of Medicine* 1981: 304; 1366

W. Shear, 'An unpleasant taste', *British Dental Journal* 1996: 180; 286

M.M. Van Ness, 'Flatulence, pathophysiology and treatment', *American Family Physician* 1985: 31; 198–200

Katherine Forrest, 'Body odour', *The Lancet* 1995: 346; 186

Murray Zimmerman, 'Unpleasant vaginal odour induced by sexual arousal', *JAMA* 1977: 237; 1735

Ken Yaegaki, 'Examination, classification and treatment of halitosis', *Journal of the Canadian Dental Association* 2000: 66; 257–61

11: THE BLADDER

P.J. Little, 'A syndrome of loin pain and haematuria', *Quarterly Journal of Medicine* 1967: 36; 253–5

R.B. Burden, 'The loin pain haematuria syndrome', *The Lancet* 1979: i; 897–900

T. Armstrong, 'Early experience of intraureteric Capsaicin infusion in loin pain haematuria syndrome', *BJU International* 2000: 85; 233–7

Editorial, 'Loin pain haematuria syndrome', *The Lancet* 1992: 340; 701–2

A.R.E. Blacklock, 'Renal autotransplantation: not necessarily a cure for loin pain/haematuria syndrome', *Journal of the Royal College of Surgeons of Edinburgh* 1999: 44; 134

Ragnar Asplund, 'The nocturnal polyuria syndrome', *Journal of Pharmacology* 1995: 26; 1203–9

Michael Lye, 'Rhythm of life and vissicitudes of old age', *The Lancet* 1999: 353; 1461

A. Mattiasson, 'Nocturia: current knowledge and future direction', *BJU International* 1999: 84S1; 33–5

W. Bromfit, 'The mysterious urethral syndrome', *British Medical Journal* 1991: 303; 1–2

Pieter Seshadri, 'Cimetidine in the treatment of interstitial cystitis', *Urology* 1994: 44; 614–16

Hans Henson, 'Interstitial cystitis and the potential role of gabapentin', *Southern Medical Journal* 2000: 93; 238–40

Magus Fall, 'Conservative management of chronic interstitial cystitis: Transcutaneous electrical nerve stimulation and transurethral resection', *Journal of Urology* 1985: 133; 774–6

12: LEGS AND FEET

J. Montplaisir, 'Restless legs syndrome: treatment with L-dopa', *Clinical Neuropharmacology* 1986: 9; 456–6

Virgilio Evidente, 'How to help patients with restless legs syndrome', *Postgraduate Medicine* 1999: 105; 59–66

Thomas Wetter, 'Restless legs and periodic leg movements in sleep syndromes', *Journal of Neurology* 1997: 244 (S1); S37–S45

Ron Pelled, 'Double evaluation of clonazepam on periodic leg movements in sleep', *Journal of Neurology, Neurosurgery and Psychiatry* 1987: 167; 1679–81

Ian Oswald, 'Sudden bodily jerks on falling asleep', *Brain* 1929: 82; 92–103

J.D. Spillane, 'Painful legs and moving toes', *Brain* 1971: 94; 541–6

A.K. Tan, 'The syndrome of painful legs and moving toes', *Singapore Medical Journal* 1996: 37; 446–7

Jeffrey Gill, 'Persisting nutritional neuropathy amongst former war prisoners', *Journal of Neurology, Neurosurgery and Psychiatry* 1982: 445; 861–5

Peter Dyck, 'Burning feet as the only manifestation of dominantly inherited sensory neuropathy', *Mayo Clin Proc* 1983: 58; 426–9

Mustafa Ertaz, 'Use of Levodopa to relieve pain from symmetrical diabetic polyneuropathy', *Pain* 1988: 75; 257–9

G. Said, 'Diabetic neuropathy: an update', *Journal of Neurology, Neurosurgery and Psychiatry* 1996: 243; 431–40

Jose Badda, 'Treatment of erythromelalgia with propranolol', *The Lancet* 1977: ii 412

M.A. Morris, 'Morton's metatarsalgia', *Clinical Orthopaedics and Related Research* 1977: 127; 203–7

Dishan Singh, 'Plantar fasciitis', *British Medical Journal* 1997 315; 172–4

14: PUZZLING PAINS

Wayne Sheils, 'Subungual glomus tumour: a cause of pain beneath the fingernail', *JAMA Georgia* 1972: 61; 268–270

Mohammad Shbeeb, 'Trochanteric bursitis', *Mayo Clinic Proc* 1996: 71; 565–9

Roger Traycoff, 'Pseudotrochanteric bursitis: differential diagnosis of a lateral hip pain', *Journal of Rheumatology* 1991: 18; 1810–12

Ilaria Merlo, 'Sciatic pain in a young sportsman', *The Lancet* 1997: 349; 846

Christine Costello, 'Vulvodynia associated with Coeliac disease', *British Journal of Obstetrics and Gynaecology* 1996: 103; 1162–3

Ahmed Shafik, 'Pudendal canal syndrome as a cause of vulvodynia', *European Journal of Obstetrics and Gynaecology* 1998: 80; 215–20

B. Ben-David, 'Gabapentin therapy for vulvodynia' *Anaesthesia and Analgesia* 1999: 89; 1459–60

15: TIREDNESS AND FATIGUE: VARIATIONS ON A THEME

Julian Stewart, 'Patterns of orthostatic intolerance: the orthostatic tachycardia syndrome and adolescent chronic fatigue', *The Journal of Paediatrics* 1989: 135; no. 2 part 1, 218–24

Frankie Campling and Michael Sharp, *Chronic Fatigue Syndrome: the Facts*, OUP 1999.

Simon Wessely, 'Fatigue syndromes: a comparison of chronic "post viral" fatigue with neuromuscular and affective disorders', *Journal of Neurology, Neurosurgery and Psychiatry* 1989: 52; 940–8

David Dawson, *Chronic Fatigue Syndrome*, Little Brown & Co 1993

Leif Solberg, 'Lassitude', *JAMA* 1984: 251; 3272–6

John Patten, *Neurological Differential Diagnosis*, Springer 1996

John Walton, 'Diffuse exercise induced muscle pain of undetermined cause relieved by verapamil', *The Lancet* 1981: I; 993

Arthur J. Hudson, 'The muscular pain – fasciculation syndrome', *Neurology* 1978: 28; 1105–9

Colin Shapiro, *ABC of Sleep Disorders*, BMJ Publications 1993

Paul Heckerling, 'Occult carbon monoxide poisoning', *The American Journal of Medicine* 1988: 84; 251–6

16: SHIVERING, HOT AND COLD SWEATS

Y. Samra, 'Dental infections as the cause of pyrexia of unknown origin', *Postgraduate Medical Journal* 1986: 62; 949–55

D.J. Eedy, 'Olfactory facial hyperhidrosis responding to amitriptylene', *Clinical & Experimental Dermatology* 1987: 12; 298–9

D.C. Seukeran, 'The use of topical glycopyrrolate in the treatment of hyperhidrosis', *Clinical & Experimental Dermatology* 1998: 23; 204–5

Abigail Arad-Cohen, 'Botulinum toxin treatment for symptomatic Frey's syndrome', *Otolaryngology – Head and Neck Surgery* 2000: 122; 237–9

James W. Lance, 'Harlequin syndrome: the sudden onset of unilateral flushing and sweating', *Journal of Neurology, Neurosurgery and Psychiatry* 1988: 51; 635–42

E. Sohar, 'Cold induced profuse sweating on back and chest', *The Lancet* 1978: II; 1073–5

17: SLEEP

Carlos Schenck, 'Rapid eye movement sleep behaviour disorder', *JAMA* 1987: 257; 1786–8

Antonio Culebras, *Clinical Handbook of Sleep Disorders*, Butterworth-Heinemann 1996

Bruce Ehrenberg, 'Sleep pathologies associated with nocturnal movement', *Movement Disorders in Neurology and Neuropsychiatry*, Blackwell Science 1999

Lee Sannella, *The Kundalini Experience*, Integral Publishing

G. Hansen, 'Schizophrenia or spiritual crisis? On "raising the Kundalini" and its diagnositic classification', *Ugeskrift fur Laeger* 1995: 157; 4360–2

R. Narayan 'Quantitive evaluation of muscle relaxation induced by Kundalini yoga', *Indian Journal of Physiology and Pharmacology* 1990: 34; 279–81

B.J. Matthews, 'Painful nocturnal penile erections associated with rapid eye movement sleep', *Sleep* 1987: 10; 184–7

18: A CLUTCH OF CURIOSITIES

P.R. Evans, 'Referred itch', *British Medical Journal* 1976 9 October: 839–41

I.W. Berman, 'Musicogenic epilepsy', *South African Medical Journal* 1981; 49–53

W.B. Matthews, 'Migrant sensory neuritis of Wartenberg' *Journal of Neurology, Neurosurgery and Psychiatry* 1983; 1–4

Dr Thomas Wehr 'Seasonal affective disorder with summer depression and winter hypomania', *Journal of Psychiatry* 1987: 144; 1602–3.

Acknowledgements

My heartfelt thanks to: Pam Dix for her major contribution to this project; Krystyna Green, Jan Chamier, Pete Duncan and Nick Robinson of Constable & Robinson; Susannah Charlton of Telegraph Books; my agent Carolyn Dawnay; and Vanessa Adams for her prodigious skills in preparing the manuscript.

This book would not have been possible without those readers of my *Daily Telegraph* column who took the trouble to write in to me with their mystery syndromes. I would like to acknowledge them here, and can only apologize for any who are left out or whose names have inadvertently been misspelled.

R. Abbott, G. Adams, K. Addis, Muriel Addison, Cynthia Ahern, Leonard Ainsworth, Penny Aitchison, L. Alexander, Anne Allen, Vivien Allen, Jacqueline Alston, M. Andrews, R. Andrews, Maureen Angell, Inge Angles, Lyall Appleby, K. Appleton, Jean Armstrong, Richard Aron, Anne Ash, Dorothy Askew, Peter Asteon, A. Astley, D. Atkin, E. Atkinson, Frances Atkinson, Maureen Atkinson, P. Atkinson, Tom Austin, Jenny Axelson, Christine Axford, H. Aylmer, Valerie Baber, Dorothy Bacon, H. Baguley, R. Bailes, Elizabeth Bailey, M. Bailey, J. Bainbridge, M. Baines, G. Baker, Stephen Baker, Yvonne Baker, Edward Baldwin, Eileen Baldwin, J. Ballantyne, Joan Ballard, D. Balme, L. Balsom, Dorothy Barber, S. Barclay, J. Barker, M. Barker, Leslie Barnard, D. Barnes, Hilary Barnes, Jill Barnes, M. Barnes, Joy Barnett, C. Barratt, P. Barrett, Richard Barron, John Bartley, John Barton, M. Barton, R.

Barton, Anne Bartram, P. Bates, Juliet Bathurst, B. Baxter, Len Baynes, S. Beatty, E. Bebbington, Margaret Bebbington, Alf Beckett, Donald Bell, Rosemary Beney, Jean Benfield, B. Bennett, Eileen Bennett, L. Benson, W. Berry, R. Bessant, Dianne Best, Dorothy Beynon, Edwin Bickerstaff, Keith Bilton, Keith Bilton, Maureen Bird, Trevor Bird, Margaret Birds, L. Birnie, R. Birts, H. Bishop, L. Bissell, M. Blackall, C. Blackburn, E. Blackburn, H. Blackwell, P. Blakey-Lodge, Walter Blanchard, Bridget Bloom, J. Blunsom, Brian Boardman, John Boden, Jane Bond, Kenneth Bone, Ken Booth, Sylvia Boregan, Bob Bottomley, Wilf Bowler, Helen Boynton, John Brace, J. Bracon, P. Braddell, D. Branch, Dorothy Brand, Edmund Brannan, Sheila Brennand, I. Brewer, M. Bridge, Jane Bridger, M. Broadbent, Norah Broadway, Derek Brocklehurst, Susan Bromhead, Ann Broomfield, C. Broucher, Alan Brown, C. Brown, Edna Brown, Isobel Brown, Molly Brown, P. Brown, S. Brown, Yvonne Brownett, Emilie Bruell, Hilary Brunyee, Peggy Brussenden, Dena Bryant, Jo-Ann Buck, G. Bucknall, D. Bukin, Mary Bull, Edward Bullen, Betty Bunce, M. Burge, C. Burgess, John Burgess, Keith Burgoyne, Angela Bursden, Jane Burton, Marion Burton, J. Burtt, P. Bush, C. Bushell, Kenneth Butler, Monica Bylte, M. Byner, M. Bysh, James Cable, Tom Caeph, Rachel Calder, Catherine Caldwell, J. Callaghan, A. Callis, Jackie Cameron, E. Campbell, J. Campbell, Robert Campbell, T. Candler, Dorothy Carlisle, Shirley Carlton, J. Carson, D. Carter, Elizabeth Carter, Joan Carter, J. Case, Fiona Cashin, L. Cassell, Dorothy Castle, C. Catellan, Marlene Cawkwell, Diana Cawson, John Cetti, Sheila Chalk, A. Chandler, M. Chandler, Nancy Chapman, Robert Chapman, Susan Chapman, Jean Chappell, G. Chatham, John Cherry, M. Cherry, Grace Chesterman, Bryan Chestle, B. Church, A. Clapham, P. Claridge, Brian Clark, Dorothy Clark, Brenda Clarke, P. Clarke, Joan Clayton, Charles Cleall, Linda Clemmit, A. Clifton, W. Coddington, Maureen Cody, Jean Cogger, D. Cohen, G. Coldham, I. Cole, M. Coleman, Monica Coles, M. Collier, Jean Collings, J. Collins, Roy Collins, Shirley Collins, M. Colville, Ann Comrade, R. Congridge, Margaret Connor, R. Cook, S. Cook, Marjorie Cooper, Pamela Cooper, Ruth Cooper, T. Cooper, B. Copp,

B. Cork, J. Cottrell, Paul Coulson, Dennis Cowen, P. Cowley, G. Cowlin, Pamela Cox, Christopher Coxon, G. Cragg, J. Cragg, Roger Cragg, J. Craig, Tony Craig, Colin Craigie, A. Crawford, B. Crawford, G. Crawley, H. Cresswell, B. Cromwell, Henry Crooks, Norah Crossley, J. Crossthwaite, Margaret Crossy, J. Crowfoot, Helen Crutchley, L. Cuff, Angela Cullidge, E. Cullin, H. Cullum, P. Cundiff, Barbara Curd, C. Currie, Rita Curtis, F. Curwood, Colin Dagnall, F. Dale, J. Dalton, Margaret Danborough, W. Dann, A. Dareucher, J. Davern, Margaret Davey, Pat Davey, Michael Davidson, Peter Davidson, S. Davidson, C. Davies, Henry Davies, J. Davies, Mary Davies, Roberta Davies, Suzanne Davies, T. Davies, V. Davies, W. Davies, Elizabeth Davison, M. Davison, K. Dawes, C. Dawson, Sheila Dawson, Jacqueline de Fomseq, A. Dean, Russell Dean, Joan Dee, J. Delaney, E. Delieb, B. Derricourt, Ann Dickinson, H. Dickinson, Anne Dickson, Kathleen Dickson, M. Dickson, Christine Dinsdale, Audrey Dix, K. Dooley, Janet Down, William Downing, Susan Druce, Howard Ducker, Eric Dudley-Smith, B. Duggleby, John Dunderdale, David Dunn, B. Durant, David Durant, Geraldine Durrant, Alan Dyson, Ina Dyson, K. Eames, Sally Earee, A. Eastham, F. Eastwood, Gwendoline Eccles, Janet Ede, H. Eirew, J. Elkington, D. Elkins, Jo Elkins, Richard Ellis, J. Evans, W. Evans, Fred Facey, Anita Falconar, John Faulkner, P. Faulkner, Moira Fenerty, W. Fenner, P. Fenson, M. Ffitch, G. Filer, W. Fisher, Anna Fletcher, Deborah Flindall, Stanley Folb, G. Forester, Gemma Forster, M. Foster, Jane Fothergill, Joseph Fox, G. Francis, Bob Frankham, C. Franklin, J. Franklin, Diana Fraser, J. Fraser, Roger Frayne, Joan Frazier, Judith Frazier, Fiona Freddi, Daphne Frost, Peter Frost, G. Froud, Maureen Frowley, Joan Fruin, Beryl Fudge, Toni Furber, W. Gadd, G. Gaillard, Paul Gallaher, W. Gardiner, D. Gatland, Helen Gazeley, Kay Geldard, R. Gentry, Elsie Geo, J. Gibson, C. Gilbert, Jennifer Goad, K. Goddard, Gwen Godfray, Donald Golden, Veronica Golding, Ruth Goldstone, Lamorna Good, W. Gooderson, Janet Goodman, C. Goodwin, Pat Gore, Elizabeth Gosling, D. Gosney, Barbara Gotts, Gillian Goudge, Glynis Goudge, Ian Graham, John Graham, Pauline Graham, A. Graham-Elwell, I. Grant-Norton, Ray Graves, Kitty Gray, R.

Greaves, A. Green, C. Green, Doreen Green, Michael Green, Veronica Green, Sarah Gretton, M. Grew, I. Grey, M. Grice, M. Griffin, D. Griffith, G. Griffiths, John Griffiths, D. Grimmett, S. Grimwood, C. Grizelle, J. Gurr, A. Gwyn Jenkins, Millicent Haberberg, D. Haddock, Barbara Hadfield, J. Hadfield, Allan Hadstone, B. Halford, Lesley Halford, E. Hall, Eileen Hall, Gerry Hall, John Hall, G. Ham, Kenneth Hammand, H. Hammond, June Hammond, Christopher Hampton, Doreen Hancock, Neil Hancox, Elizabeth Hardaram, D. Hardisty, Wendy Harie, Ann Harland, M. Harris, Pat Harris, Walter Harris, Alan Harrison, Edgar Harrison, Joyce Harrison, D. Hart, E. Hatch, E. Hatley, G. Hatton, J. Hawes, F. Hawkins, A. Hawkrigg, Kathleen Haworth, J. Hayle, Dorothy Hayward, L. Hayward, John Hazeldine, R. Hearnden, M. Heasman, Joyce Heath, Mary Hedley, J. Heilbronn, Brian Henderson, G. Henderson, Joy Hennah, John Henton, P. Heppenstall, Anne Heselton, M. Hesford, E. Hewison, Celia Heyburn, J. Heyburn, Harry Heywood, Mary Hibbs, J. Hickling, B. Hicks, Eileen Hicks, J. Hill, R. Hill, Peter Hills, M. Hindmarsh, Faith Hines, M. Hird, A. Hiscock, A. Hoath, Kathleen Hockey, Heather Hodgett, Bill Hodgson, A. Hodson, M. Hoek, Angela Hoffmann de Visme, June Hogarth, Lesley Hoggard, P. Holderness, Olive Holkham, F. Holland, Geoffrey Holmes, G. Hood, Violet Hopwood, Sue Horbert, Marian Horner, Marian Horner, Robin Horseman, C. Hoskins, Debbie Hoult, R. House, Elisabeth Howard, W. Howarth, Valerie Howdle, M. Howell, Betty Howlett, Frank Hoyle, M. Hryniewicz, Jean Hubbard, A. Hughes, D. Hughes, G. Hughes, I. Hughes, Peter Hughes, V. Hughes, D. Humphrey, C. Humphrys, E. Hunt, J. Hunt, John Hunt, Naomi Hunt, S. Hunt, Elisabeth Hunter, J. Hunter, Evan Huntington, G. Hutton, L. Hutton, I. Iberson, David Iliffe, Eric Ingham, N. Ingram, V. Jack, H. Jackman, K. Jacques, Sarah James, M. Jannetta, M. Jarrett, Susan Jarvis, Carol Jeavons, M. Jeffrey, R. Jenkins, Robert Jenkinson, Paul Jennings, Suzanne Jennings, Barbara John, A. Johnson, E. Johnson, Ernie Johnson, Gillian Johnson, Iris Johnson, Lynda Johnson, Michael Johnson, Pam Johnson, Audrey Johnson, H. Johnston, Helen Johnstone, D. Jones, Gareth Jones, Nigel Jones, Patricia Jones, Peter Jones, Shirlie

Jones, E. Josh, Sylvia Kaines, O. Kaye, Beryl Keane, H. Keightley-Hanson, V. Kelly, R. Kempton, G. Kenderdine-Davies, Kathryn Kent, I. Kerrell, Evelyn Keys, Colin Kidd, J. Kilby, Julia Killey, John King, W. King, Maureen Kirby, Jean Kirkland, Veronica Kirton, Jennifer Kitley, Ellen Knight, R. Knight, T. Konwerski, William La Chenal, Dee Lacey, R. Ladd, Adrian Lambert, Barbara Lambert, David Lambeth, J. Lamont, Dorothy Lane, Wendy Lane-Davies, Barbara Langley, C. Langley, Pauline Langley, Hugh Lantos, Mary Larrett, Sheila Laughton, Yvonne Lauter, Ian Lavery, Jane Lavington Evans, Margaret Lawrence, R. Lawrie, W. Leadbeater, K. Lean, John Leane, Janet Lee, Pamela Lee, Robert Legg, Doreen Leigh, Margaret Leighton, Kathleen Lemman, A. Leng, J. Lennard, F. Leonard, Y. Leuridan, J. Levene, Anthea Levene, Richard Lewcock, Andrew Lewis, C. Lewis, O. Lewis, Paul Lewis, Valerie Lewis, R. Linden-Kelly, Gemma Lindon-Travers, A. Lloyd, Annabel Lloyd, D. Lloyd, J. Lloyd, Elisabeth Lockhart, J. Logan, Teresa Lonergan, G. Long, R. Long, J. Longden, Josie Loosemore, Megan Lovegrove, Mary Lovemore, Patricia Lowe, A. Lowther-Pinkerton, Jim Ludlow, Duncan Lunan, J. Lunnon, R. Lyon, Anne Macaulay, D. Macaulay, Angus MacDonald, Ian Macdonald, V. Macdougall, Derek Mack , Susan Mackellar, B. Mackie, P. Mackinnie, M. Mackintosh, Roderick Mackley, Kathleen MacKrill, P. Maclachlan, Margaret Maher, Jean Maish, Brenda Mallett, L. Manktelow, David Manley, A. Mann, Sylvia Mann, D. Manning, Donald Manson, Adrian March, D. Marchant, Jacqueline Marle, E. Marot, V. Marriner, J. Marriott, Marion Marriott, Paul Marshall, Marion Marshall, Jane Marston, Elizabeth Martin, M. Martin, Ruth Martyr, B. Mason, Felicity Mawson, W. Maycock, Douglas McCord, H. McGill, K. McGrath, Field McIntyre, Margaret McIntyre, J. McKellow, P. McKeown, Carol McLean, J. McNally, A. McWilliam, Betty Mears, Jean Medcalf, V. Mellon, E. Mellor, Ann Mellors, Diana Menzies, Rosemary Menzies, Lysbeth Merrifeld, Frances Michels, John Miles, Judith Miles, Douglas Millar, Gillian Miller, Susan Miller, E. Millett, Elizabeth Mills, C. Milner, B. Mingham, D. Minor, D. Minterns, Micky Mitchell, Sally Mitchell, Sylvia Moffatt, John Monnington, Patrick Montgomery, Karen Montini, A. Moody, Bernard Moret, F. Morgan, M. Morgan, Patricia Morris, Colin Morse, Patricia Morse, Fiona Morton, A. Mould, J. Mountford, Gill Mullings, Joan Murray, Judith Muston, Antony Narula, B. Naylor, Margaret Naylor, Caroline Neat, Patricia Nelson, Margaret Nevard, Richard Neve, L. Neville, C. Nevins, David Newman, Kenneth Newton, Fergus Nicholson, D. Nickols, J. Nickson, J. Nickson, Charles Noble, Victoria Nock, Sandy Nokes, Kate Norbury, Beryl Norton, Anne-Marie Nowell, M. Nowers, Margaret Nye, Patrick O'Keeffe, Paul O'Neill, J. Oakford, Barbara Oakley, Josephine Oakley, Elizabeth Oats, M. Olive, Elizabeth Oliver, Jean Oliver, Paul Oliver-Smith, Dorothy Organ, M. Ormerod, Margaret Ormonde, Hugh Orr, J. Owen, Joan Packham, Barbara Paddon, Joan Palmer, Bettine Panes, J. Parker, M. Parker, S. Parker, G. Parkinson, Charles Parlett, M. Parnell, P. Parr, E. Patchett, T. Paulley, Michael Payne, Anne Pearce, V. Pearcy, Jeffrey Pearson, Hylda Peart, Edgar Peel, James Peel, Janet Perry, Donald Pettet, David Pettle, Madeline Phillips, Guy Pilbeam, Doreen Pill, Pamela Pineo, Mary Pink, P. Pinnington, John Pinnock, Rhona Pisani, Tony Platts, B. Pledger, Jean Plesked, Kenneth Polkinghorne, Vivienne Polley, Benjamin Portmoy, Hilary Potts, Margaret Pottter, Janet Powell, Betty Praill, Diana Price, V. Price, S. Prior, A. Pryer, Trevor Pugh, John Pughe-Jones, A. Pulbrook, Zilvia Pumfrey, D. Queripel, Margaret Quin, David Rabone, G. Ragoni, Pat Rand, Marie Randall, M. Ransom, J. Rattray, R. Raven, E. Rawlings, Penelope Rawlinson, Hazel Rea, M. Redrup, R. Reed, D. Rees, Kathleen Reilly, Don Richards, John Rickard, Marianne Rigge, Keith Ripley, F. Ripper, June Risden, W. Robbins, G. Roberts, I. Roberts, J. Roberts, Julia Roberts, A. Robertson, J. Robertson, R. Robertson, Edmond Robinson, Edna Robinson, Kathleen Robinson, S. Robinson, William Rodley, H. Rogers, R. Rooney, G. Rose, J. Roseman, G. Ross, K. Rowe, Victor Rowe, Stanley Rubin, Derek Rudden, M. Rundle, Susan Russell, Patricia Ryrie, Neville Sadler, Hilda Sager, Heather Salmon, G. Salter, David Salvage, Valerie Salzen, Karen Sammuell, Diana Samways, Marilyn Sandy, K. Sansom, D. Savage, D. Sayer, Charles Scandrett, E. Scanlon, Mary Schofield, Elizabeth Scoble-Hodgins, A. Scott, F. Scott, Jan Scott, P. Scripps,

Peter Seaby, L. Seatter, M. Seymour, Helen Shaffner, K. Sharp, John Shaw, Margaret Sheaf, Helen Sheen, J. Shergold, M. Sherratt, Frances Shilston, Jane Sholl, B. Shuker, C. Shulman, M. Siddall, Gloria Siggins, Glenys Simkins, M. Simmons, E. Simonis, E. Simpson, W. Simpson, Eileen Sinclair, Leslie Slade, Nicola Sly, Ann Smallman, Charlotte Smallwood, Debbie Smeed, A. Smeeton, Judith Smethurst, Betty Smith, Denis Smith, E. Smith, F. Smith, Henry Smith, Lynette Smith, Mary Smith, Peter Smith, R. Smith, Una Smith, V. Smithson, William Smurthwaite, Barbara Sobey, Rosie Somers, Robin Somes, Molly Spence, Judith Spurgeon, L. Spurring, John Squire, Patricia Sreeves, Ivy Stafford, M. Stammers, Peter Standbridge, G. Staniforth, B. Stapleford, Barbara Stapleton, J. Stay, Margaret Steele, J. Steen, Anthony Stephens, R. Stephenson, David Stevens, Joan Stevenson, Ian Stewart, Jenny Stobart, J. Storm, I. Strachan, V. Streten, G. Stubbs, D. Sullivan, Edna Summergood, Jessie Summers, A. Sumner, J. Sumner, G. Sutherland, K. Sutherland, Frank Sutton, Gillian Swan, J. Swanbrow, Mark Symons, R. Taionis, Basil Tait, Inge Tait, Lynda Tanfield, Mary Tapsford, M. Tay, C. Taylor, E. Taylor, Hazel Taylor, Jean Taylor, John Taylor, Paul Taylor, E. Tedcastle, Mark Ter-Berg, Eric Thomas, K. Thomas, A. Thompson, G. Thompson, Gwen Thompson, Robina Thompson, Sheila Thompson, W. Thompson, Elaine Thomson, Mary Thomson, Betty Thomson, H. Thundow, Jan Timson, Richard Tinson, C. Tomkins, Garth Tomlinson, Thelma Toms, E. Towns, Annie Townsend, Molly Townson, Carolyn Trainor, Daphne Trake, Patricia Travis, Mary Trumpess, G. Tudor, Maureen Tupholme, H. Turkington, G. Turner, Margaret Turner, J. Turney, Bob Turvey, Marjorie Twitchett, C. Twynam, Peggy Tyler, Jill Tylet, J. Tyrrell, G. Tyte, K. Underwood, John Unsworth, P. Unwin, R. Unwin, Beatrice Urquhart, Norman Van Abbe, Giles Van Colle, Alan Varle, John Varley, A. Venn, Nick Violaris, J. Visser, R. Waddington, Trevor Waddon, H. Wale, G. Walker, Mavis Walker, C. Wallace, J. Wallace, C. Wallden, R. Walrond, Audrey Walsh, S. Walsh, Sheila Walsh, Alan Wanstall, Elizabeth Ward, John Ward, Mary Ward, P. Ward, Christopher Warner, Pauline Watford, F. Watkinson, G. Watkinson, J. Watson, Augusta Watts, Katie Watts, D. Wattson, K. Weatherley, D. Webb,

Daphne Webber, Lorraine Webdale, Fin Webster, Margaret Webster, Daphne Wedgbury, D. Weight, H. Welbourn, G. Wells, A. Werran, Ralph Werrell, John Weston, Isobel Whatrup, Sue Wheadon, Joan Wheatley, J. Wheeldon, P. Whiffen, Kenneth White, Roger White, B. Whitechurch, Peter Whiteley, Jenny Whiteside, John Whittle, L. Wibbam, Hilda Wickes, Rex Wilcox, Sheila Wilcox, M. Wilder, Marguerite Wilkins, Hazel Wilkinson, Betty Wilks, Mark Wilks, Karen Willcock, D. Williams, Laura Williams, M. Williams, S. Williams, Tony Williams, R. Willison, John Willoughby, D. Wilson, M. Winder, Daphne Windsor, John Winkler, E. Winterborn, Murray Withers, H. Witt, Maria Wood, P. Wood, J. Woodall, Shirley Woodall, Barbara Wooddisse, Joan Woodward, C. Woolnough, Susan Wormale, Joan Wormleighton, Audrey Wright, David Wright, John Wright, W. Wright, Stephen Wyllie, Patricia Yates and Martin Young.

Index

Other titles available from Robinson Publishing

The Family   Foreword by James Le Fanu   £9.99 [ ]
Encyclopedia of
Medicine & Health
Answers all your questions about health today in a way you really understand, including up-to-date findings on vaccination and new sections on keyhole surgery, screening, palliative therapy and antenatal diagrams.

The Complete Guide   Pamela Brooks   £9.99 [ ]
to Allergies   Introduction by Dr Sarah Brewer
Comprehensive, practical, up-to-date and jargon-free, for everyone who has ever suffered themselves, or has a child or other family member who suffers from an allergic reaction.

Chronic Pain   Arthur C. Klein   £7.99 [ ]
                      Foreword by Dr James Le Fanu
Based on the experiences of the *real* experts – people with chronic pain who have found a way back to full and active lives.

How to Live to 90   Dr James Le Fanu   £7.99 [ ]
Once past the watershed of their 50th birthday, most people will turn their attention to extending their chances of a long and healthy life – but where to start?

Robinson books are available from all good bookshops or can be ordered direct from the Publisher. Just tick the title you want and fill in the form below.

TBS Direct
Colchester Road, Frating Green, Colchester, Essex CO7 7DW
Tel: +44 (0) 1206 255777   Fax: +44 (0) 1206 255914
Email: sales@tbs-ltd.co.uk

UK/BFPO customers please allow £1.00 for p&p for the first book, plus 50p for the second, plus 30p for each additional book up to a maximum charge of £3.00.

Overseas customers (inc. Ireland), please allow £2.00 for the first book, plus £1.00 for the second, plus 50p for each additional book.

Please send me the titles ticked above.

NAME (block letters)..

ADDRESS ....

....

.... POSTCODE ....

I enclose a cheque/PO (payable to TBS Direct) for ....
I wish to pay by Switch/Credit card

Number ....

Card Expiry Date ....

Switch Issue Number ....